# Caring ar

*Caring and Coping* provides a clear and accessible explanation of the history, politics, management, funding and day-to-day work of the social services in Britain.

Social care now encompasses a wide range of increasingly specialised professions. *Caring and Coping* aims to improve the student's, the practitioner's and the general public's understanding not only of what these various professions do, but also what the legal, political, ethical and financial constraints are upon them. It succinctly addresses issues such as the terms and effects of the Children Act and the NHS and Community Care Act, the place of charities in the modern welfare state, the role of management, relationships with other agencies, and the place of social work within the community.

Social services are so often portrayed in the media in a sensationalist way and this book counterbalances the hype by referring to solid research and a more down-to-earth picture. It is therefore an ideal introductory text for those training to be social workers, as well as the interested layperson.

**Anthony Douglas** is Director of Social Services, London Borough of Havering and **Terry Philpot** is editor of *Community Care*.

# Caring and coping

## A guide to social services

Anthony Douglas and Terry Philpot

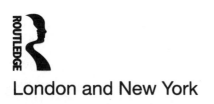

London and New York

First published 1998
by Routledge
11 New Fetter Lane, London EC4P 4EE

Simultaneously published in the USA and Canada
by Routledge
29 West 35th Street, New York, NY 10001

© 1998 Anthony Douglas and Terry Philpot

Typeset in Times by Routledge
Printed and bound in Great Britain by Creative Print and Design
(Wales), Ebbw Vale

*British Library Cataloguing in Publication Data*
A catalogue record for this book is available from the British Library

*Library of Congress Cataloguing in Publication Data*
Douglas, Anthony
Caring and coping : a guide to social services / Anthony Douglas and
Terry Philpot.
Includes bibliographical references and index.
1. Social service – Great Britain. 2. Human sevices – Great Britain –
Management. 3. Caregivers – Great Britain. I. Philpot, Terry. II. Title.
HV245.P49                                                         1988
97-32824
361.941–dc21                                                      CIP

ISBN 0–415–16032–4 (hbk)
ISBN 0–415–16033–2 (pbk)

*To Margaret, Sarah and Gemma Douglas*
*and – again, as he deserves it so – Robert Philpot*

# Contents

# Authors

**Anthony Douglas** is Director of Social Services, London Borough of Havering. He was previously Assistant Director of Social Services, London Borough of Hackney and has also worked in the London boroughs of Southwark, Barnet and Newham. He has been an adviser on major studies like the Audit Commission's *Misspent Youth* and is a member of the executive council of the Association of Directors of Social Services and of its children and families committee. He is an advisor to the Local Government Association. He has written and lectured extensively on social services. Before entering social work he was an economist and a journalist.

**Terry Philpot** is editor, *Community Care*. He has edited a number of books, the most recent of which are (with Chris Hanvey) *Sweet Charity: The Role and Workings of Voluntary Organisations* (Routledge, 1996) and *Practising Social Work* (Routledge, 1993), and (with Linda Ward) *Values and Visions: Changing Ideas in Services for People with Learning Difficulties* (Butterworth-Heinemann, 1995). He is also the author of *Action For Children* (Lion, 1994). He was made an honorary member of the council of the NSPCC in 1991 and has won several awards for journalism. In 1990 he was granted a British Council fellowship to look at services for people with learning difficulties in Czechoslovakia.

# Foreword

The need for a book which explains the history, politics, management and the day-to-day work of social services – 'the fourth arm of the welfare state', in the words of one no less than Stephen Dorrell, the last Conservative Secretary of State for Health – in a readable style for a wide audience has long been apparent. There are several good books aimed at social policy students but few, if any, which seek to inform students (including social work students), the general public and practitioners and managers in social care.

But why is this book intended not only for students but also for the last two groups? As to the general public, most people do not come into contact with social workers in the way that they have dealings with doctors, the police or teachers. And for many of those who do, it is not always a welcome experience: social workers try to help and support but they also have wide-ranging powers to intervene in family life.

But even the way in which the jobs of those who work within social care are described is far from being self-explanatory. What do social workers do? As long ago as 1978 Barbara Wootton could write of recruitment advertising for social workers:

> one such [advertisement] asks for applicants who are used to 'statutory duties' and the ability to 'act independently and take appropriate decisions' (about what?). Another mentions that the successful applicant will be expected to 'work with families and children' (on what?) and yet another asks for an 'intake social worker' to 'join a team' which is 'developing systems and methods useful to clients and staff'. The layman may well be puzzled to visualise how the holders of these posts will spend

their working hours. Yet he would have no similar difficulty in describing a day in the life of, say, a doctor or a school teacher.

(Wootton 1978)[1]

Our belief also is that, with regard to the general public, too often newspapers carry stories about the latest child abuse scandal, where blame is often apportioned for some shortcoming on the part of social workers. Or there are court cases about children abused in children's homes by those who care for them. Or a random murder by a mentally ill person throws a harsh spotlight on the supposed shortcomings of care in the community policies in which social services departments play a critical role. All too often such stories only leave the general reader, at best, bewildered and, at worst, thinking that 'the system' – whatever that may be – has failed.

Yes, there have been failures by individual workers and management and supervision systems. But what such stories all too often lack is a context. What are social services? How have they emerged? Who runs them and manages them? Who funds them? What role do politicians, locally and nationally, play? What is the difference between the public and voluntary sectors? What training is available to those who work in both sectors, and to whom are practitioners and those who manage them accountable? And, to use Barbara Wootton's phrase, how do social workers spend their working hours?

Our hope is that this book will answer those and many other questions which the intelligent, concerned but often confused member of the public will ask. As to our wish to interest those who (unlike social work and social policy students) already work within the social services, the system of social care in this country has fragmented in the last ten to fifteen years for both professional and political reasons. Professionally, workers have come to specialise more and more. Thus someone working in child protection may have only the most basic (if that) understanding of, say, care of elderly people or working with people with learning difficulties. Services have fragmented, too, in a number of other ways, largely through political pressures. The voluntary and private sectors now play a much greater part in providing services. The split between those who purchase and those who provide services has caused another divide both between those sectors and within social services and social work departments. In addition, a whole culture of managerialism has grown up populated by many whom, some would argue, have but the slightest connection with day-to-day practice.

We hope, therefore, that this book will serve as a bridge between these various outposts of the vast empire which is now social care, enabling those who soldier therein, at whatever level, to have a greater understanding not only of what their colleagues do but what the legal, political, philosophical and financial constraints upon them are.

Two other points need to be made. The first is that while Wales has, like Scotland, voted for devolution, the legal and local government systems of Wales and England remain broadly similar. Services in Scotland and Northern Ireland, however, have very different histories and reasons why they have developed as they have, which has resulted in different legislation, legal systems and systems of local government. It would have been tiresome for the reader to be constantly reminded that while a certain point was true for England and Wales, there was a significant difference in Northern Ireland or Scotland. Thus, we have included a chapter devoted to the particular differences in those two countries.

The second point is that we have tried as far as possible to explain various concepts such as the purchaser/provider split or the provisions of various pieces of legislation or ideas like 'needs-led assessment' and 'user-led' services. We have not taken for granted that all this is familiar to the reader. While we have used cross-references, we have not assumed that the book will be read as a whole but accepted that readers may wish to choose chapters of interest to them. Nor do we assume that an explanation in only one chapter is sufficient for it not to be mentioned again in another. Thus, to do this it has been necessary to include some repetition which we hope will not interfere with the flow of the text.

Anthony Douglas wrote Chapters 2, 3, 4, 5, 8, 9, 10 and 12 and Terry Philpot wrote Chapters 1, 6, 7, 11 and 13. Both authors would like to express their gratitude to Polly Neate, managing editor of *Community Care*, who kindly read the whole manuscript in a very short space of time and made a number of incisive comments and suggestions, which have improved the final product immensely. In addition, we would like to thank Bob Holman, community worker in Easterhouse, Glasgow, and a prolific author in his own right, for reading Chapters 1 and 13 and making many helpful suggestions. Des Kelly, Human Resources Director, Care First, read Chapter 7 and Quintin Oliver, Director of the Northern Ireland

Council of Voluntary Action, also read Chapter 13. Our gratitude to all of them is gratefully acknowledged here. None of the above, of course, are responsible for the opinions contained herein, which remain the authors' responsibility.

Finally, our families put up with long hours devoted to writing this book. Their support and forebearance were crucial.

Anthony Douglas and Terry Philpot
London and Surrey
April 1998

# Introduction

Social services helps millions of people but, paradoxically, millions more know nothing much about them. Social services' responsibilities are awesome. They cover fostering, adoption, child protection, children needing care, mental health, people with dementia, frail elderly people, disability, youth crime, drug abuse and alcohol abuse, to mention just a few. While social services is not a 999 service, it operates round-the-clock providing crisis services, short-term support and long-term care.

Social services has to make sure that vulnerable people in Britain are protected and supported. Their responsibilities are clearly defined in law, particularly by the Children Act 1989 (implemented October 1991), and the NHS and Community Care Act 1990 (implemented April 1993). Along with health care, education and income support, social services and other welfare agencies are the basic building blocks of a civilised society.

Either the state, the family, the community, the employer, or a combination of these, are responsible for a nation's social services. In the UK, the state has been a near monopoly provider of welfare since 1945. There are signs of a shift in this country towards placing more responsibility with the family or with social services users, either through increased charges for services or through private insurance schemes. Indeed, insurance companies are focusing on welfare as a significant future growth area in their strategic plans. In some East Asian states, the responsibilities of the community and the employer are more important, with businesses continuing to provide many welfare services for their employees, although economic pressures in the new tiger economies coupled with an ageing population are leading to increases in state care. In a number of European countries like France and Germany, children are legally obliged to contribute financially to the costs of the long-term care of their parents. The situation in the UK will inevitably change. At the time of the Beveridge Report in 1942 which launched the British welfare state, there was 1 pensioner for every 5 people of working age. By 2030 there will be 3 for every 5. Whatever the mix of insurance and higher taxes, working people will pay more towards both their own care and the care of future generations of pensioners without means.

Good health care, decent housing, education and income support are also part of a comprehensive approach to welfare. Services which need to be brought together for maximum effect remain largely unco-ordinated. Fragmentation has characterised both central and local government. There is often a muddle inside central government about policy direction, and a desperate bid to avoid high spending, leading to policies which in fact 'dump' vulnerable (and expensive) groups on other departments. There is tension at the local level between departments in the same council about which services warrant a higher corporate priority in budget rounds. Warily tolerated both centrally and locally, social services also symbolises national mixed feelings about any further growth in welfare-related budgets.

Policy confusion becomes more important to sort out because of deteriorating social conditions for many British families in the 1990s. In fact, 1 in 3 children in the UK live in poverty, according to a study by the European Union statistics agency Eurostat, partly because the gap between rich and poor has been widening since the mid-1970s. The need for welfare provision is closely linked to poverty, deprivation and social class, although of course being poor and deprived does not automatically lead to other problems. Although social evils such as child abuse cross classes and cultures, the bulk of welfare concerns centre on poor people. The probation service deals with one-tenth of the unemployed people in the UK. As already disadvantaged people grow poorer, so the pressure on social services increases to cover gaps arising elsewhere in the welfare system. If it is to mean much in the twenty-first century, the British welfare state will need to be reinvented, as the percentage of national income spent on public services expenditure dips below 40 per cent. Even with cutbacks in other European countries, Germany, France and Italy continue to spend over 50 per cent of their national income on public services. In Britain, the status of social services as a Cinderella public service seems guaranteed.

While a minority of British citizens can buy their way out of trouble, most people living in Britain may need social services at some point in their life, either for themselves, for someone they care for, or for someone who is in some way dependent upon them. That might be an elderly relative going downhill fast with dementia, a child with a disability, a sister trying to adopt for whom a character reference is requested, a teenage child in trouble with the police, or a close friend addicted to hard drugs or alcohol. These are mostly eventualities we hope won't happen to us, and each problem is usually just as difficult to resolve for professional staff as the person or family directly involved.

In practice, social services is rarely the source of support for the average person up and down the country. While GPs are more likely to be consulted about major life crises, social workers are not, except in a handful of extreme cases by people who already know and use the system or are forced into it. UK citizens suffer alone, supported by an invisible army of unpaid carers – relatives, friends, colleagues at work, voluntary groups, churches and neighbours. Apart from anything else, welfare state professionals are in extremely short supply. Ironically, they in turn look for back-up from the same invisible army.

How does social services affect the average person? You may be invited to comment on a planning application to establish a hostel for people with mental health problems near where you live. You have read about high-profile murders committed by young men with schizophrenia who should have stayed in hospital. You do not want dangerous ex-patients on your doorstep. You may also have seen an elderly person living in appalling conditions of self-neglect and feel angry that 'they' seem to allow this. 'They' normally means social services. This book tries to explain why certain social services decisions are made.

The welfare state has lost its way. From its conception in 1945 until the mid-1970s, it attracted cross-party political support and steady growth. The International Monetary Fund crisis in 1976 was a watershed. From then on, each new government decided the share of national wealth devoted to public expenditure had to be reduced. Globalisation and international competition also increase economic pressures and the marginalisation of people inside each country who make little contribution to the national economy, and who in fact draw resources from it. For social services nationally, needs have been growing faster than the resources allocated to meet them.

Rationing is now universal. On top of that, Conservative administrations between 1979 and 1997 tried to alter the relationship between the state and the individual so that individuals had more responsibilities than rights. Weakened by this Darwinian approach to social policy, in which the glorification of the fittest accompanied the maligning of the weakest, the notion of caring for others was subtly replaced by a notion that needing help is faintly immoral. Social exclusion replaced social care, although this in itself was not new. Social exclusion has a long and infamous history.

Economic pressures are limiting the affordability of state care around the world. Britain is said to be following the United States in social trends and policy. The re-emergence of a hard-line approach in the USA augurs poorly for Britain. In 1996, the US Congress passed the Personal Responsibility and Work Opportunity Act, under which 'absolute' limits can be set on the amount of welfare benefits a person can receive in his or her lifetime.

In August 1997, the *New York Times*[1] reported that benefits to 100,000 disabled children, one-tenth of the total number receiving them, and over half of the initial review sample, had been cut off as a direct result of the new welfare law. After a forty year break, chain gangs are back inside prisons in southern states like Alabama. Groups of over twenty prisoners are shackled together working the fields and the local Interstates, supervised by guards with rifles. The policy is popular, but is regarded by its critics as heralding a return to a vicious racist past as 75 per cent of the prison population are black. Removal of social security benefits and zero tolerance of crime are social policies which risk hardening the attitudes and behaviour of society's underclass.

This book looks at what the future holds for social services and considers how continued public expenditure pressures and the ageing population in particular might be managed. This is another area of social services provision which affects many people, particularly sons and daughters who feel deprived of their rightful inheritance if the bulk of their parents' assets and life savings are claimed by local authorities to help pay for care the family regards as a right.

It is thus no surprise that the decisions and competence of the staff delivering these services are questioned. It is also not surprising when social issues raise such disquiet that society looks for someone to blame when mistakes are made, especially in serious child care cases. Social workers top many people's lists of pet hate figures, often through a misunderstanding of their roles, and a lack of awareness of the legislation they have to administer. In children's homes, some of the most damaged and difficult young people in the country are looked after by badly paid, unqualified staff. It would be surprising if there weren't problems. Experienced practitioners are often promoted to be supervisors and managers, leaving the most inexperienced staff on the front line to deal with the public. Public scrutiny of social services is higher now than it has ever been, yet the lay person's views are often formed by media coverage of cases that go badly wrong, which give an unduly negative overall impression because they are not representative. This book seeks to increase lay awareness of social services without covering up professional shortcomings.

Times have changed. There were seven social workers for children in Oxfordshire in the 1960s: now there are more than a hundred. Taking the second half of the twentieth century overall, social services have expanded beyond the wildest dreams of early visionaries. But changes in culture lag well behind. When one of us was growing up, in a London suburb in the 1950s, a residential home for people with learning difficulties opened in the next street. It was known locally as 'the Spastics place'. Residents, when they were allowed out, which wasn't a lot, were laughed at. Children crossed the road to pass by on the other side, mimicking their movements.

In those days, adopted children were called bastards, and the word 'illegitimate' had a common currency. That was the 1950s. It wasn't until 1978 that the first person with learning difficulties passed the driving test. In 1997, in the London borough where one of us works, on Guy Fawkes night, a group of boys and girls aged about 13 surrounded a man with learning difficulties at a bus stop in broad daylight and put a lit firework into his trouser pocket. The man was burnt and developed nightmares, losing all confidence as a result. As we approach the year 2000, we have to ask ourselves how much has really changed.

# Chapter 1

# From charity to social work
## A history

A time traveller to the classical world would find himself or herself able to call on the services of an engineer, architect, lawyer and doctor. Social work is a latecomer among the professions (if, indeed, it can be called a profession at all). It emerged, fitfully, from the tide of nineteenth-century philanthropy and then largely as a voluntary activity, often undertaken by women. Social work is a product of industrialised, urban societies, dealing with the personal consequences of social dislocation. And while Britain is one of the societies in which it can earliest be identified as a discrete activity, its forms differ from society to society according to the political and social culture and historical traditions.

## ORIGINS OF SOCIAL WORK

In the UK social work has developed, within a century, from its primitive, philanthropic origins to a highly professionalised activity undertaken (or at least overseen) by large public sector agencies. It is not difficult still to detect its beginnings – Dr Barnardo's, The National Children's Home and Orphanage (the present-day NCH Action For Children) and the NSPCC, are only three of the charitable organisations with their roots in Victorian philanthropy and social concern. Yet today they continue with large professional staffs, offering often unique services, while also sometimes mirroring local authority activity, when not actually working in partnerships with local councils or even directly funded by them.

Residential care, in particular, derived from the successive Poor Laws of the last century. Only now have we wrested ourselves from the grip of the large-scale institutions which became an increasingly prominent feature of state provision from the seventeenth century for children and the physically disabled, the mentally ill, elderly people and people with learning difficulties (Parker 1988), and (with the Poor Law Amendment Act 1834) the poor. That latter legislation is popularly credited with having introduced the ideas of 'deserving' and 'undeserving poor' as a criterion for the receipt of relief (assistance). But while this was so as a legal concept in the seventeenth century, some charities would not help the children of single mothers. With the weight of such historical and cultural baggage, it is not difficult to see how, particularly after 1979, the concepts of 'deserving' and 'undeserving' were revived in attitudes towards unemployed people and some other groups like single parents (mainly mothers) and asylum seekers. However, as Parker points out (1990), unlike in England and Wales, there was no Poor Law relief in Scotland available for the able-bodied and there was, therefore, no necessity to create a workhouse system to test the eligibility of applicants.

Social work's origins lie in concern for the relief of poverty and destitution and (in the case of children and prostitutes) with the idea of 'rescue'. Its first practitioners tended to be middle class and conservative, often inspired by Christian ideals but uninformed by any secure knowledge base. Marxism lacked much impact, while sociology was in its nascent stages and the influence of psychology non-existent. Along the way social work has, magpie-like, collected a knowledge base, borrowing from psychological and sociological insight, with a dash of political radicalism thrown in, but without developing much distinctive knowledge of its own.

The early pioneers developed their work and social work methods largely through working with children (most prominent among them Thomas Barnardo, Edward Rudolf of the Church of England Central Home for Waifs and Strays – now The Children's Society – and Thomas Bowman Stephenson of the National Children's Home) and the poor. 'The poor' was an umbrella term which covered many groups with whom social workers were later to specialise – families, elderly people, and those with physical, mental and learning difficulties.

For many social workers the newly developing sociological findings of people like Charles Booth tied in with their own wish to understand why those with whom they worked behaved as they did and also to discover the potential numbers with whom they could work. Octavia Hill, Helen Bosanquet and Charles Loch, the founders of the Charity Organisation Society (COS) (and Octavia

Hill in her work in providing housing for the poor), and Canon and Mrs Barnett, of Toynbee Hall Settlement, London, began systematic record keeping. It was not just knowledge which they required but usable knowledge (Younghusband 1981). They (and the founders of the child care charities) tended to work with the individual, to want to develop character, to 'rescue' them from corrupting social and family environments, which often meant getting them away from drink and prostitution and making them employable. There was much emphasis on the supposed moral deficiencies: drunkenness, fecklessness and sexual licence on the part of parents (Philpot 1994a). As Alfred Majer, one of Stephenson's collaborators, wrote, with regard to the emigration policies which saw tens of thousands of British children, poor, orphaned and abandoned, sent to the colonies:

> The town-bred youth in his teens – the flabby, discontented, restless juvenile product of pavement and poverty must be weaned from the glare and the glitter, the vice and the unwholesome excitement of our streets. His habits must be steadied and renovated by a course of systematic industry, upon the land, if possible, miles from 'the madding crowd's ignoble strife'.
>
> (Bradfield 1913)

Such a philosophy applied not only to the emigration policies undertaken by the Home, Barnardo's and other societies, but to the removal of children from their environment and families to homes elsewhere in this country.

One consequence of the emphasis on work with individuals was the development of casework, the earliest social work method, pioneered by the Charity Organisation Society (Younghusband 1981). However, Frank Prochaska suggests that casework had earlier origins than the COS, showing that it emerged from the work of Mrs Ellen Raynard's Bible and Domestic Female Mission, founded in 1857 (Prochaska 1990). In essence, the method was to discover the relevant facts about the client and their situation, make a plan with them, and give help adequate to meet whatever their needs were perceived to be.

The COS was primarily concerned with material need, preventing pauperism, eliminating handouts and encouraging thrift. Strongly moralistic, it adopted wholeheartedly Poor Law notions of 'deserving' and 'undeserving'. It saw those with whom it came in contact with as the 'helpable' and 'unhelpable' (Younghusband

1981). The former were those who were, with assistance and moral fibre, able to surmount crises and become law-abiding and industrious. The unhelpable fell into two groups: those who were feckless and irredeemable and those whose condition was due to mental or physical frailty or illness or old age. The latter did not require casework but medical care or financial help. But for none of them would Octavia Hill and her fellow founders of the COS countenance old age pensions, state benefits or school meals. The work of charity, the support of friends, relatives and neighbours was enough to bring a life of prudence and thrift to those who could attain it. Anything else was to encourage pauperism and undermine the incentive for honest work.

In the 1950s and 1960s casework came to mean supporting the person to help them seek insight into problems and effect a permanent change. It was a view by then strongly influenced by psychoanalysis and particularly the views and work of Donald Winnicott, the child psychiatrist, and Clare Winnicott, who headed the child care course at the London School of Economics. Casework was less concerned with external influences on individuals like poor housing or money problems. As casework grew in modern times it came to include liaising with other agencies with whom the client – not yet the 'service user' – had a problem, and the giving of advice on matters like welfare benefit entitlements. But casework was to come under attack from radical elements within social work. What has now become community work and group work had its origins, in part, in the work of the university settlements (most notably, those in Birmingham and Liverpool and the work of the Barnetts at Toynbee Hall) with emphasis on group discussions, activities, outings and parties and a small number of members to each helper. Barnardo and Bowman Stephenson, while concerned with individual children and unafraid of seeing moral defects in those with whom they worked, nevertheless also provided collective provision, as well as the homes which they built for their children to live in. Both began workshops for boys to learn trades. Barnardo turned a gin palace into a coffee palace, akin to today's community centre, and Stephenson founded a cripples parlour, which was his equivalent to the modern day centre.

Bowman Stephenson and Barnardo were among the first to see that children were not best cared for in large institutions. Both placed emphasis on the children living in small homes under the care of houseparents, who were often married couples (the cottage system) (see Philpot 1994a and Wagner 1979).

As well as these pioneers there was also the work of the Salvation Army (founded in 1879 after William Booth had set up the East End Revival Society in 1865, which he later renamed the Christian Mission) to assist social casualties and the police court missioners of the Church of England Temperance Society (who later became the contemporary probation officers). In 1895 the first hospital almoner (social worker) was appointed.

## SOCIAL WORK IN THE TWENTIETH CENTURY

Perhaps social work's comparatively swift birth and rapid growth in the latter part of the last century exhausted it. Certainly, in the first half of this century there was little activity. A debate was occasioned by Beatrice Webb's dissent from the report of the Royal Commission on the Poor Laws, which reported in 1909. Sidney Webb was not a member of the commission but it is believed that he wrote much of the minority report, which Beatrice and others signed. Their view was diametrically opposed to that of Hill and her COS colleagues (the majority report was drafted by C. S. Loch, then secretary of the COS) – the deterrent effect of the Poor law did not work; charity could not be seen as a solution to widespread poverty, unemployment and destitution. The solutions of the COS (and, indeed, of social work generally) could not overcome low wages, sweat shops, long working hours, slum landlords and the complacent rich and supine local authorities. Collective action, not charity or casework, was the answer. Social services should ensure an optimum minimum condition of life. 'Interfere, interfere, interfere', said Sidney Webb (Jones 1972). The surveys of Seebohm Rowntree and Charles Booth gave statistical evidence to what all but those who were ideologically hidebound could see with their own eyes. Booth's reports had begun to appear in 1883. They showed not the existence of a 'submerged tenth' but that 35 per cent of the population had only the barest necessities to get by on, and 9 per cent had less than the minimum (Booth 1902).

The Independent Labour Party was founded in 1893 and the Labour Representation Committee (the first parliamentary grouping of Labour MPs) was formed in 1900. Great changes were brought about after the radical Liberal Government won a landslide victory at the polls in 1906: old age pensions were introduced, along with progressive income tax and labour exchanges. There were trade boards with powers to fix wages and hours in sweated industries. There were benefits for the sick, the unemployed and the widowed. National insurance was introduced. Juvenile courts and protection for neglected children came into being, as did better public health provision.

Most of this left social work on the margins. Beatrice Webb had seen that 'the naughty boy, the homeless and neglected child, the unhappily married, the neurotic invalid are clearly not problems in isolation but, partly at least, the products of the problems of some home' (Cormack 1953). Eileen Younghusband summed up social work's failure which led to its isolation at this period:

> The creative pioneers had somehow failed to disentangle social work as a relevant form of practice to meet social need from an outmoded ideology. And when they themselves retired or died, no second generation of leaders attuned with the times but with their force and zest, indeed their influence in the corridors of power, succeeded them.
>
> (Younghusband 1981)

The clouds were not entirely without a break. The Probation of Offenders Act 1907 permitted (and then required under the Criminal Justice Act 1925) probation officers to 'advise, assist and befriend' those given probation. Almoners were employed in voluntary and municipal hospitals. Psychiatric social work came into being, with the development of the insights afforded by the knowledge of psychiatry, and psychiatric social workers were often employed within child guidance clinics which grew in number in Britain in the 1930s. But probation officers, almoners and some psychiatric social workers were employed in agencies whose primary purpose and professional expertise were not social work. Most social workers were employed in voluntary agencies and many of them were doing relief work. When they were not caring for children, they were undertaking the work that Hill and her colleagues had mapped out for them decades before.

The Second World War changed all that. The welfare of children was the motor which drove reform. The war years had inculcated a greater public consciousness about children deprived of family life. A perceived need of the British army for physically strong young men also lay behind welfare provision such as free milk and free school meals. Thousands of children – often from the poorer, city areas and children who were in residential care – had been evacuated from their homes to places of greater safety (Holman 1995). People who before had been unaware of the plight of many children and the conditions in which they lived and had certainly never known what it was like to live in a residential home, found billeted upon them children who suffered the pain of separation from brothers, sisters, parents and others who cared for them. It was not only the general public who were learning from this experience. Those who were professionally concerned with children – social workers, psychologists, civil servants – began to learn new lessons about the effects of separation and loss. The lessons learned by trained social workers who were employed in the evacuation centres were to prove invaluable when they found themselves working, only a few years later, in the new children's departments.

There are certain times when circumstances coincide to make radical change possible. Even during the war, the reforming Education Act was passed in 1944 and a Minister for Reconstruction had been appointed to the Cabinet to look beyond the cessation of hostilities. As the war drew to an end and as the concerns about evacuated children grew, albeit inchoately, two events conspired to give substance to these concerns, to point the way forward and to draw social work out of the shadows and allow it to share in the coming social change. In May 1944 Lady Allen of Hurtwood wrote a letter to *The Times* expressing her concern about 'children who because of their family misfortune find themselves under the guardianship of a Government Department or one of the many charitable organisations' (Allen 1944). She went on to refer to

> many thousands of children [who] are being brought up under repressive conditions that are generations out of date and are unworthy of our traditional care for children. Many who are orphaned, destitute or neglected still live under the chilly stigma of 'charity'.
>
> (ibid.)

Staff, she added, were 'for the most part overworked, unpaid and untrained'. She criticised the lack of supervision in the training system and inadequate supervision and inspection.

The letter provoked an enormous correspondence in the newspaper's columns. Six months later Lady Allen returned to the fray, substantiating her claims in a pamphlet, *Whose Children?* (Allen 1945). We do not know what the effect of all this agitation might have been had that been all. But a second event occurred which made the movement for change irresistible.

In January 1945 the inquest took place into the death of Dennis O'Neill, a 13-year-old boy who had been starved and beaten to death by his foster father in a remote farmhouse in Shropshire, where he had been placed by Newport Borough Council. The inquest jury made its criticisms and an inquiry under Sir Walter Monckton was set up. He criticised both Shropshire County Council and Newport for their failure to supervise the placement. But the government also set up, under Miss Myra Curtis, a committee of inquiry to look at the care of children 'deprived of normal home life with their parents or relatives'. It was empowered to discover what should be done to 'ensure that these children are brought up under conditions best calculated to compensate for the lack of parental care'.

The committee interpreted its brief liberally – destitute children, those who were homeless, children awaiting adoption, those believed not to be educable or with a psychiatric disorder, children who were physically disabled or who had a learning difficulty, children orphaned as a result of the war: the condition and needs of all children were considered. Among other things the committee found

> a widespread and deplorable shortage of the right kind of staff, personally qualified and trained to provide the child with a substitute home background. The result in many [residential] homes was a lack of personal interest and affection for the children which we found shocking. The child in these homes was not recognised as an individual with his rights and possessions, his own life to live and his own contribution to offer.
>
> (Curtis Committee 1946)

Too often, it went on, children's homes were characterised by 'dirt and dreariness, drabness and over-regimentation'.

While Curtis believed that voluntary agencies should 'continue their present activities in the care of children', it also called for a wholesale reform of children's services at local authority level. The Children Act 1948 was based directly on the recommendations of the report and its main provision was to create in each local authority a children's department, staffed by child care officers (social workers) who were under a children's officer. A number of other changes stemmed from the Act, not least the great boost which it gave to fostering. Curtis had believed that fostering or adoption (adoption was legalised in 1926) should be the preferred option and children's homes were to be secondary to this. The Act said that fostering should have priority unless this was 'not practicable or desirable for the time being'. Finding foster homes, screening applicants, making satisfactory placements and supervising them allowed social workers to develop new expertise.

Contemporary with Curtis in England was the Clyde Committee in Scotland. It, too, reported in 1946. It argued strongly in favour of fostering as 'the nearest approximation to family life'. After that it favoured small children's homes. Nearly 18,000 children were in the care of five statutory bodies in Scotland (voluntary agencies looked after nearly another 5,000). The committee believed it 'inappropriate to leave these children in the hands of a Public Assistance Authority with a Poor Law outlook'. It proposed, therefore, that a new local authority committee be created to look exclusively after the welfare of deprived children (Holman 1995). Unusually, while there were two reports, Curtis and Clyde, in the three countries, England and Wales, and Scotland, one piece of legislation, the Children Act 1948, heralded reform across the borders.

As for voluntary agencies, in the inter-war years they continued to grow but to offer more of what they provided rather than innovations. Certainly, in the case of the big child care charities, the 'orphanage' became a standard form of provision at this time. This was so even for what was now the National Children's Home and Barnardo's, whose founders had pioneered different, more family-orientated forms of residential care. Voluntary agencies did come to pioneer new methods of working in the 1960s and 1970s with, for example, young offenders and families. But it was not until the 1980s that a new, larger and more powerful role was allotted to them with the coming of new community care legislation and the move away from local authorities as providers, as opposed to purchasers, of services (see Chapters 3 and 5).

From 1945 to 1979 Labour and Conservative governments came and went but these were the years of post-war consensus. The Tory party accepted the welfare reforms of the post-war Labour Government and the differences in the following years tended to be marginal rather than fundamental. This was the face of politics in so far as it affected social work. Within social work there were debates about its direction, even, from a radical wing, its very *raison d'être* – were social workers necessary? Did they hinder rather than help? Could they claim to help when they were agents of the state? Didn't the poor require money and not counselling or casework?

The disenchantment with established thinking, as seen in the student disturbances of the late 1960s, was expressed in social work with the influence of the anti-psychiatry movement of R. D. Laing and Thomas Szasz. If psychiatry was a 'con', a means of control, so was social work practised as casework. (The radical social workers' magazine, which exercised some influence at one time, was entitled *Case Con*.) 'Radical social work' had its high point in the 1970s. Its primary objection to casework was that casework saw problems rooted in individual and personal failure rather than the wider social problems of unemployment, poor housing and poverty. Casework was thought actively to inhibit the client from understanding the structural inequalities that were at the root of their problems. Radical social workers castigated those who favoured casework as 'social policemen', a means of social control and radical social workers aligned themselves with general political radicalism.

But the attacks by radical social work did not kill off casework. There were, of course, some social work clients who did have personal problems not related to material conditions. Also, there were those who argued that some other forms called social work were not social work. Community workers, for example, objected to being called social workers. Indeed, in 1982 Robert Pinker, in his dissenting note to the Barclay Committee, which looked at the task and roles of social workers (Barclay Committee 1982), declared unequivocally that 'social work is case work' (Pinker 1982).

In addition, the casework of the 1950s and 1960s underwent a change in that it came to embrace feminist counselling in relation to rape and domestic violence, advocacy and advice work. It is also the fact that is arguable that in the 1990s casework emerged in a different guise as care management; or perhaps it is truer to say that there are strong elements of casework to be found in care management (see Chapters 3, 5 and 6).

Social work no longer has the self-confidence to engage in such debates at a time when it lacks political and public support. One product of its lack of self-confidence is that inwardly it has been self-castigating and outwardly it has lacked a voice. Social work is also now more modest about what it can achieve. There have been some lastingly beneficial results of 1960s' activism which have flowered in the late 1980s and 1990s. One of these has been the user movement, the belief that clients have rights and skills and can contribute to a more effective service (see Chapter 6). Radical social work has not been responsible for this alone but it has played a major part in forging a path. Likewise, the focus on anti-racism and gender issues as they affect clients and professionals has also emerged from that radical period.

But whatever criticisms radicals might make of social work during this period it enjoyed a higher status and esteem then than it had before or since. Greater public expectations and the increased demand for services were matched by greater resources. Expenditure on the personal social services had been static in the 1950s but doubled between 1960 and 1968 (Adams 1996). Juvenile crime rose and there was a larger population of elderly and physically disabled people. In the late 1960s Enoch Powell, then Minister of Health, made a speech about 'making a bonfire' of the long-stay institutions, thus provoking an early intimation of the policy of community care. Attitudes to certain groups underwent a positive change and social work threw off the last remnants of its judgemental attitudes.

There were no more reorganisations of local government at this time (in vast contrast to the continuing upheavals of the next twenty-five years). Thus time, money and energies were spent on service development. But there were several pieces of legislation which affected social workers and enhanced their role – from the emphasis on preventive work to work with juvenile offenders or those at risk of coming into conflict with the law.

The professional self-confidence of social work was so strong that it played a key role in what was to be the most important reform since those under the Children Act 1948. Despite all the advantages which the latter had brought social workers employed in the public services, they were still employed in three separate local government departments: children's, mental health and welfare. When the government established the Seebohm Committee it made its brief 'to review the organisation and responsibilities of the local authority personal social services in England and Wales' (Committee on Local Authority and Allied Personal Social Services 1968).

The report believed that a unified social services department was needed. But it also attributed to the new departments ambitions which even at the time may have seemed grandiose and later came to seem delusional. The report stated:

We recommend a new local authority department, providing a community-based and family-orientated service, which will be available to all. This new department will, we believe, reach far beyond the discovery and rescue of social casualties; it will enable the greatest possible number of individuals to act reciprocally, giving and receiving service for the well-being of the whole community.

Following the report's recommendations, the Local Authority Social Services Act 1970 created the comprehensive, powerful social services department, into which were subsumed the three departments, to provide a 'community-based and family-orientated' service (ibid.). Seebohm had explained that 'we could only make sense of our task by considering also childless couples and individuals without any close relatives; in other words, everybody'. Universal services, not just for the poor but for everyone, would be offered, in Seebohm's phrase, 'through one door on which to knock'. The era of stigma (it was supposed) was past.

The reforms which the Seebohm Committee was to recommend were broadly similar to those put forward by a three-person working party set up by the Secretary of State for Scotland and the result was the creation in Scotland of social work departments. However, the Social Work (Scotland) Act 1968 was more all-inclusive than the English and Welsh legislation (see Chapter 13).

The Seebohm reforms all but coincided with the massive reorganisation of local government. In 1974, three years after they were created, social services departments found a new home with the reformed local authorities. The numbers of staff increased, departments spread their wings, services were enhanced, there was greater funding and a new, longer managerial ladder was created. Importantly, there were gains in the coherence, planning and delivery of social services (Adams 1996). And in the year that the new departments came into being, the Certificate of Qualification in Social Work, the first general (as opposed to specialist) training for social workers, was introduced.

Social work's standing increased but it was not without controversy. Seebohm had envisaged generic social services, which came to be interpreted as generic social work. Thus, social workers began working with all manner of clients at the cost of their long-perfected specialisms. It took many years for specialism to come back into fashion and, arguably, not without loss to client care, particularly that of children and mentally ill people.

But the honeymoon created by the birth of new departments did not last long. The death of Maria Colwell in 1973 and the consequent outcry were the beginning of public and political disenchantment with social work's role and the loss of its own self-confidence. The subsequent inquiry into her death proved to be the first of many; many of which would come to the same conclusions and make the same recommendations. Perhaps, most significantly, it took child abuse to the top of the social work agenda, affecting the shape of services and, to an extent, the allocation of resources thereafter.

But one other event at the end of the decade had widespread repercussions for social work and social services departments. In May 1979 Margaret Thatcher was swept to power as the head of the new Conservative Government. Here again was the reformists' hour, although they were reforms of a very different kind from the liberal ones which had gone before. There were several consequences of the Conservatives' 18-year hegemony.

First, Seebohm had envisaged a universal service, a kind of welfare version of the National Health Service. This was somewhat optimistic anyway. Social services had long been plagued by – and, under the new organisational arrangements, continued to be plagued by – stigma, and to say that one had been to see one's social worker was not the same as saying one had been to see one's GP. The Labour Governments which preceded those of Thatcher and John Major had made inroads into a universalist approach to welfare by charging for some services and the effects of deepening unemployment threw more people into the welfare net. But the scythe of change cut far deeper under the Tories. Often social services are the place of last resort – for the troubled child, the abusive parent, those whom the other public services cannot or will not assist. Schorr (1992) makes the point:

> The most striking characteristics that clients of the personal social services have in common are poverty and deprivation. Often this is not mentioned, possibly because the social services are said to be based on universalistic principles. Still, everyone in the business knows it. One survey after another shows that clients are unemployed, or to observe a technical distinction, not employed – that is, not working and not seeking work. Perhaps

half receive income support, as many as 80 per cent have incomes at or below income support levels.

But, second, there were other changes which the Conservatives made which, directly or indirectly, had their impact upon social workers and their departments – these were policies on juvenile justice, social security, child support, housing and asylum seekers, and a wholesale reform of the NHS.

But none had such a fundamental impact as the reforms, enshrined in the National Health Service and Community Care Act 1990, which shook up social services departments themselves. These reforms, in part, stemmed directly from the disenchantment with public services which had been partly responsible for the Conservatives' election victory.

There were strong financial reasons underpinning the reforms (see Chapters 5 and 6). But the creation of the so-called mixed economy of care, which meant that the voluntary and private sectors would have a much greater part in providing services, and the introduction of market disciplines gave a new role for social services departments and, arguably, changed social work more fundamentally than had the Seebohm reforms. Social services departments ceased to be 'monopoly' providers of care. Whole parts of their empires, particularly in the residential sector (see Chapter 7), were shed. Responsibilities which had seemed formerly to be securely theirs were contracted out. In many parts of the country – though not all, this was one of the problems in trying to stimulate a market of care – new providers of services mushroomed and long-established ones, particularly the big voluntary agencies, radically reshaped themselves to compete for custom. With the advent of the care manager the essence and distinctiveness of social work itself were brought into question. Voices were raised which announced the imminent death of social work.

In the years of reform, from the Children Act 1948 through to the immediate years of the Seebohm reforms, social work, in Younghusband's phrase (Younghusband 1978), 'leapt from the margins to the centre'. One of the curious effects of the Conservative reforms of public services in the 1990s was to make social services departments the largest and biggest spending local authority departments (curious because the Conservatives seemed to find social work and social services departments temperamentally unpalatable). But the irony was that for all the status that departments have come to enjoy in collaboration with colleagues in the police, education and the NHS, and for all the variety of work which fell to them – from arranging adoptions to working with elderly people – social services still works almost entirely with people on the margins.

But to look here at what social services do with and for the people with whom they work, the ways in which work is carried out, and the impact that that has had on the profession and standing of social work would be to pre-empt much of the rest of this book, which deals not with the past but with the uneasy present and the uncertain future.

# Chapter 2

# On the statute book
## The law and social services

Social services staff absorb general legal principles but rarely familiarise themselves with the fine print or with research findings. It would help if they did. For example, a study by Marsh and Triseliotis in 1996 found that the average social worker thought that only 25 per cent of children returned home after a period in short-term care.[1] The real figure is over 90 per cent. Basic social work is too often poorly informed.

In the early to mid-1990s, over 100 volumes of new government guidance on social care were issued, much of it structuring social work at a national level for the first time. Clear standards were set. Although this amounted to a sea change in communication about what government expected social services staff to do, it was by and large written in a way that sent social workers to sleep, and has had a limited impact on what they actually do on the ground, with a few plainly written and well-illustrated exceptions, such as Joyce Plotnikoff and Richard Woolfson's *Reporting to Court under the Children Act*.[2] The unfortunate truth is that despite the best efforts of managers and trainers, the influences on social work practice are more personal and diverse. External influence in the form of supervision and training may change what someone does by 20–30 per cent at most.

While the legal framework for social services only changes once in a few decades, new case law is being made all the time, much of it requiring changes in policy and practice. The law is a general expression of the way society is moving, the guidance gives the law a push in a particular direction, then everyone waits for judges to clarify what it means in practice.

Social services decisions tend to remain invisible because the people they support are unlikely to make a fuss. In recent years, a number of lawyers representing service users have instituted proceedings seeking to establish precisely what local authorities have a duty to pay for. Cases can take years to resolve. It is a recipe for continuous uncertainty about the true extent of local authority social services departments' powers and duties. Taking local authorities to court is vital to opening up decision-making, but it may also make local authorities more cautious and rule-bound. Two young adults, having lost their cases in British courts, are taking cases to the European Court against local authorities who they claim should have taken them into care to prevent them being subsequently abused at home. Since the early 1980s, when Graham Gaskin, who had been in care in Liverpool, took his local council to court for refusing to let him see his case records, a succession of children have sought retrospective justice against damage allegedly done to them in care. In 1998, ten people with learning disabilities were awarded £800 compensation each when it was found they had been refused service in their local pub in Loughborough two years before. Case law can be a great force for civil rights.

Case law has become popularly known by the names of the local authorities who bring or defend a particular action. The Gloucestershire judgement, reached in 1996, stipulated that local authorities cannot use resource shortages as a reason for refusing to provide the community care services a disabled person has been assessed as needing. This Court of Appeal judgement was subsequently overturned in 1997 by the House of Lords in a 3–2 vote, which then established the reverse principle: that resources can after all be taken into account. Meanwhile, the Lancashire judgement said that where a need has been assessed, a local authority is entitled to provide for that need in the cheapest possible way, even if the service user wants a more expensive service, as long as the need is being met. These cases illustrate how a confusing patchwork of decisions determines how billions of pounds of public money are spent.

The Oldham judgement determined that a court had the power to direct a local authority to assess a family in a residential family centre of the court's choice, rather than the local authority having the final say on where and how to carry out the assessment. Residential family centres cost up to £2,000 per week per family, and are not subject to any formal inspection and registration process which protect standards of care, so the judgement carried major implications.

Initially, Sefton Council successfully argued it should be able to dictate the level of savings a person who has been funding their own residential or nursing care could retain before the local authority starts to pick up the bill. The law stated that at least £10,000 of a person's savings or capital are immune from being used for this purpose, but Sefton set the threshold at the cost of a funeral – around £1,500. The Court of Appeal later reversed this decision, and set a binding principle that £10,000 of a person's assets are after all immune. At the time of writing, Sefton Council has an appeal pending in the House of Lords. The legal battleground these days is as much about resources as professional issues. The last Conservative Government recognised this as early as 1992 when through the Social Services Inspectorate it wrote to all local authorities advising them not to place on record 'unmet need', in order to protect themselves from legal challenges if they couldn't afford to pay for services.

Tower Hamlets Council was told it must re-assess an 11-year-old boy's housing situation to see if it fell within the general duties set out in the Children Act. That judgement has major implications and implies a possible return to the 1950s and 1960s, when social services did take children into care if they were living in poor housing or their parents were homeless. The 1966 TV drama *Cathy Come Home*, and campaigning organisations like Shelter, led to changes in housing law which put a stop to all that, but social policy changes are always potentially reversible.

Case law can also be contradictory. While some recent judgements have recognised that resource shortages clearly limit what can be provided, others give new rights to people with no reference to resource implications. In June 1997, a deaf nursery nurse, Becky Halliday, won a case in the House of Lords against Peter Lilley, the last Social Security Secretary of the Conservative Government. The judgement stated that the care component of the Disability Living Allowance benefit could and should cover needs beyond a basic subsistence level. Lilley argued that the benefit should only cover essentials. The judges agreed with Becky Halliday, who wanted to pay for a sign language interpreter, that claimants should be able to live 'reasonably' and that a 'reasonable' lifestyle at least extended to paying for an interpreter. The so-called 'Wednesbury' principle established many years ago that local authority decisions must above all else be reasonable.

General social services responsibilities are set out in the 1970

Local Authority Social Services Act, and these have not changed significantly in twenty-five years. However, the ways in which they are discharged have changed fundamentally. While there are between fifty and a hundred separate Acts of Parliament setting out specific social services responsibilities, the main laws cover children's services, community care for elderly and disabled people, mental health services, youth crime and the registration and inspection of residential homes.

## THE CHILDREN ACT 1989

Implemented in 1991, the Children Act was a unifying piece of legislation, updating all past children's legislation which had accumulated piecemeal from 1933 onwards. The cornerstone of the legislation was its emphasis on the welfare of the child as the prime consideration, asserting this principle as greater than all others. The accompanying guidance also stressed the need for social services to work in partnership with parents. The principle of 'parental responsibility' was introduced, which also covered private law cases such as divorce and separation. Across the spectrum, parents' views were to be deemed, in theory at least, less important than what was objectively best for their children, whose wishes and feelings had to be formally taken into account in all decisions made. Parents would never lose their share of parental responsibility, even when their children were in care. Responsibility and accountability rather than sheer power were highlighted. The 'no order principle' meant that all positive alternatives to a court order must be explored first. Powers to remove children from home in an emergency were strengthened by the replacement of the old Place of Safety Order with a new Emergency Protection Order. A new Child Assessment Order was brought in, and a Specific Issues Order, which covered one-off issues where a legal decision was needed. A new Residence Order made it easier for relatives or foster carers looking after children to obtain security both for the child they looked after and themselves. Services to under-8s, like playgroups, childminders, nursery schools, nursery classes and private nurseries, were to be formally reviewed every three years.

The Children Act can also be seen as part of a wider international movement, in Europe, the USA and Australia and New Zealand at least, towards asserting the rights of children. A new complaints and representations procedure was introduced as part of the Children Act. The United Nations Convention on the Rights of the Child has received general endorsement by child care organisations in the UK. Campaigns have been mounted by many of the same organisations to establish a children's commissioner, along the lines of the ombudsman, or a minister for children. However, by 1997, the situation some children and young people found themselves in had worsened, if empowerment assumes access to resources. For young people needing to set themselves up independently, after abuse or neglect at home, where their suffering had not been disclosed to anyone, their prospects were grim. Changes in income support rules mean hardly any 16 or 17 year olds now qualify for food and rent payments. Changes in housing benefit rules mean that young people are only eligible for housing benefit in restricted circumstances. While one arm of government spoke about children as citizens with rights and responsibilities, other departments suggested they should live at home until they were earning sufficiently to set up home on their own, leaving no exit route apart from the street for young people unable to cope with serious family conflict and disturbance. The Labour Government of 1997 ruled out the idea of a minister for children. The laws protecting children are still not tight enough. For example, there are no checks made on the carers of children subject to Residence Orders in private law proceedings. In two cases in Tameside in 1996, sex offenders were able to secure Residence Orders on children because no social worker or guardian *ad litem* had been appointed to check into their background.

## THE CRIMINAL JUSTICE ACT 1991

This Act replaced juvenile courts with youth courts, and subsequent guidance introduced national standards for the supervision of offenders.[3] The Children Act had replaced previous legislative provision which allowed young people who committed offences to be put in care by a juvenile court. From this point on, care issues were to be dealt with by new family proceedings courts. Separating out issues of care and control was not easy, and the debate continues to this day as to whether youth crime is best handled within a punitive framework, or by early intervention using family support approaches.

The 1991 Act also made provision for video recordings of children who either said they had been abused, or who professionals thought had been abused, to be shown in an adult court as part of a criminal trial. This prevented direct intimidation in court of a victim by an abuser, at least while the victim gave their own evidence. Interviews with children had to be conducted within a framework set out in the *Memorandum of Good Practice*, which advised against leading questions, or in any way contravening principles of total neutrality in the preparation of children for an interview, and in the conduct of the interview.[4] As some of the case studies set out in Chapter 4 and Chapter 12 show, the rights of defendants to a fair trial and to the protection of their civil liberties may still be valued more highly than the rights of children to be protected at all costs.

## THE NHS AND COMMUNITY CARE ACT 1990

The NHS and Community Care Act, phased in between 1991 and 1994, has transformed health and social services to people over 18 in a number of ways. For the first time, the views and needs of users were to be organised through a process called commissioning. This was distinct from the views of service providers about what was best for users. The distinction is more than semantic. For the first time, users had to be consulted legally about which services they prefer. Historically, their views had at times been overlooked by a culture of 'the professional knows best'.

For some service users, new ways of communicating had to be found. In Somerset, for example, the Somerset Total Communication Project was set up by Somerset County Council to gauge the wishes of people with severe learning difficulties, whose views were often submerged by the louder views expressed by their parents and carers that they would be best off living in residential care. When consulted, people with learning difficulties invariably want to live in small homely settings with one or two other people, which after all is what most of us want! This process of user involvement has been radical in social services, and has set off a number of tensions between new commissioning staff, whose job it is to seek the views of service users, and providers, many of whom have vested interests in maintaining current types of provision.

Assessments are the primary legal basis for service provision. For example, Section 47 of the NHS and Community Care Act 1990 places a duty on local authorities to 'assess those who may be in need of community care services and decide whether those services shall be provided'. The Children Act places exactly the same onus on local authorities in respect of children in need. Assessments range from risk assessments of children in their family, of how dangerous to himself and others someone with a severe mental health problem might be, to functional assessments of an elderly person's ability to carry out basic household and personal care tasks. To carry out an assessment, the person doing the assessment will need to gather information about the social and personal circumstances of the person needing help, and to interview both the person and anyone else who has vital information before coming to an informed judgement. While there are any number of check lists to assist assessors, much of the information is capable of more than one interpretation, hence the single most important factor is professional judgement.

The conclusion of each assessment should be set out in a care plan, which is then put into practice by a care manager. Care managers update and monitor care plans, sometimes along with 'provider co-ordinators' or 'care co-ordinators' who work out the fine detail of daily care programmes. Care plans should be reviewed at least every six months, and much more frequently if a person's situation is volatile. To be effective, care should be organised and managed across agencies from a single co-ordinating point. Care management is carried out by social workers or other community care professionals such as home care organisers or district nurses. While it does not matter from which professional group a care manager is drawn, it is essential the role of care management is seen as a purchasing and commissioning role, built around the concept of a needs-led service. This is important if the care manager was previously a provider, like an occupational therapist or indeed a home care organiser. Care managers have to divorce themselves from provider interests, not just commercial interests, but from a certain way of rigid professional thinking which ex-local authority providers may still retain from the old municipal days. The skills required for successful care management are broader than traditional social work skills and include the commissioning of resources and purchasing services within an agreed budget, as well as old-style social work skills like counselling and carer support.

Several American managed care programmes, such as On Lok (meaning a peaceful happy abode), which operates in San Francisco's Chinatown, organise all health and social care services for an individual from a single funding stream. The programme covers long-term care in the community. On Lok has its own day care and respite care provision, so it is both a purchaser and provider.

We have mentioned 'purchaser (or commissioner)' and 'provider' already. They are key terms. The principle is that assessors (or purchasers or commissioners), acting on behalf of service users, should be free to buy services from the provider whose services best meet a particular need. In practice, the social care market took a while to take off, but taken off it has, and there is now far more choice of services available. Some local authorities no longer provide any residential care services, purely acting as purchasers or commissioners. Others, either for political or geographical reasons, or because their own provision is the best available, have retained some direct provision like home care services, day centres and residential homes.

Commissioning is the term used for deciding which social care services should be purchased and developed. In joint commissioning, one or more agencies commission and specify services together. This has conventionally been social services and the local health authority, but the process can be extended to include other agencies controlling funds like local education authorities. Intelligent commissioning accepts that more needs-led services will inevitably mean that a greater mix of service providers are required to cater for highly specialised needs, but it does not make the mistake of determining the commissioning mix ideologically. Intelligent commissioning matches services to needs, irrespective of who provides them.

By contrast, commissioning myopia only looks at one agency at a time, and only looks at one way of doing things rather than appraising alternatives. Commissioners have to look to the future and assess the impact of wider influences on the social care market. A new minimum wage in the first term of the current Labour Government will push up private sector prices, but then local authority costs will also be pushed up by the new single status pay and grading framework. It is always difficult making cost comparisons between local authority provision and private home provision, because the dependency levels of residents can vary between the two sectors. It is more sensible for managers of residential services to monitor their own costs and ensure good value for money or 'best value' through self-regulation.

Commissioning is usually carried out in relation to localities or areas with a population between 150,000 and half a million. The largest authorities commission for populations over a million, while some GP 'total fundholders' commission for less than 10,000 patients. Commissioning care rationally across lop-sided structures and populations is unnecessarily complicated. For example, Wales has five health authorities and twenty-two local authorities. Proposals on co-terminosity made in the 1998 NHS White Paper, 'The New NHS', should improve the effectiveness of joint planning.

Between 1993 and 1998, 85 per cent of each local authority's government grant for new community care services had to be spent in the independent sector. The independent social care sector is growing fast, like local authority social services departments did in the 1970s when they were first set up. It is a market in which the smaller suppliers are being swallowed up and squeezed out by the big boys, including American and European consortia who are rapidly diversifying into different types of provision, like any other expanding business. For example, Care First is a private care business formed through a merger between two of the largest private care companies, Court Cavendish and Takare. Apart from direct provision of its own, Care First now runs local authority homes for a number of authorities including seven homes for the London Borough of Bromley and fourteen homes for Bedfordshire. This would have been unthinkable fifteen years ago. Their size also enables them to cover short-term losses in any one unit, and thereby to provide smaller specialist care homes such as a small unit for Parkinson's disease sufferers. Because local authorities are not allowed to borrow capital in the way the private sector can, only private sector providers can meet modern design standards for care homes. Medium-sized and large businesses can also absorb short-term revenue losses, as profit margins running a care home invariably come from selling the last one or two beds, and going from 95 per cent to 100 per cent occupancy.

Although the NHS and Community Care Act set out a clear framework for the assessment and planning of community care needs, it said little about who would be eligible for direct care services, so old legislation going back to the 1948 National Assistance Act still applies. Old laws used a different language and were written in a different time. Clever lawyers can drive a coach and horses through the gaps. The 1970 Chronically Sick and

Disabled Persons Act is still used as the legal benchmark of what resources have to be provided to a disabled person, and the gap between what the 1970 Act can be interpreted as meaning and what the 1990 Act says is fertile territory for lawyers and advocates. Unifying legislation such as a Community Care (Consolidation) Act is needed to make the situation clearer, especially about baseline entitlements. The NHS and Community Care Act also let health and housing authorities off the hook, by shying away from making their involvement in community care service assessments and provision mandatory.

The Act led to other profound changes and improvements. It forced all but a small number of renegade local authorities to upgrade their dismal and unfit old people's homes to modern design standards by 1998. Rather than 90-year-old strangers sharing a room as if they were in prison, residents could start to expect decent-sized, well-fitted single rooms. Some homes are now like classy hotels, with facilities such as en suite bathrooms, licensed bars, hairdressing and organised entertainment. Some local authorities were forced through the financial regime at the time to transfer their residential homes to the independent sector in order to meet the cost of refurbishments. Most set up not-for-profit trusts, transferring all their staff into third party organisations. Some authorities closed residential homes altogether and built new sheltered housing to a high standard into which residents transferred, becoming tenants rather than residents in the process, although some lawyers took the view that providing sheltered housing and round-the-clock care still fell within the definition of a residential care home. The distinction was important because tenancies cost local authorities less than residential care, and left the tenants with more money in their pockets because of added social security benefits, than the personal allowance or 'pocket money for grown ups' that they previously had received as residents of care homes. A variety of housing associations and consortia gradually became involved in the provision of care, thus meeting one government objective of creating a so-called 'mixed economy of care', where a range of independent providers would be encouraged to enter the social care market.

# THE MENTAL HEALTH ACT 1983

The Mental Health Act is now nearly fifteen years old, although an accompanying code of practice has been revised on a number of occasions, the latest edition coming out in 1997. It sets out the types of assessment needed before psychiatrists and social workers can detain and treat someone in a psychiatric unit against their wishes. This power to lock up someone who is mentally ill is colloquially called 'sectioning', which refers to the various sections of the Mental Health Act under which someone can be detained. Periods of detention vary from a 'Section 5 (2)', which allows a registered nurse to detain a patient in hospital for a matter of hours only, through a 'Section 4' (for a 3-day maximum period), a 'Section 2' (for a 28-day maximum for the purpose of assessment), and then finally a 'Section 3' (for a 6-month maximum to allow for treatment, but only if the patient is defined as 'treatable', which excludes a lot of people who pose an equal threat to themselves or others). A rarely used power of guardianship allows a local authority to compel an adult to receive specified community care services. The rights of patients are defined, especially rights of appeal against detention and treatment. With hindsight, the most important section of the Act turned out to be a small section on the services to be arranged once someone has left hospital, known as 'after care', Section 117, which places a responsibility on health and social services to devise a care plan for anybody with mental health problems discharged back into the community from hospital. When things go wrong, the lack of a clear care plan, or the fact that it wasn't implemented, is often the reason. The Act started with much more of a focus on the rights of patients. Now it is the rights of the public to protection from a small group of potentially violent schizophrenic patients which are topical. The 1995 Mental Health Patients in the Community Act tightened up the supervisory requirements, possibly as a stepping stone to a new Compulsory Community Treatment Order. Local supervision registers of patients at greatest risk are also in force, but are rarely used with any conviction, as practitioners feel they do not assist them with the crucial issue of compulsory treatment, and access to secure in-patient beds.

## THE REGISTERED HOMES ACT 1984

The Registered Homes Act sets out the requirements and standards which must be met by private or voluntary residential care homes with more than four adult residents. An amendment in 1991 introduced modified regulations for homes with fewer than four residents. Under this Act, the responsibilities of the owners of homes are defined, the suitability of the individual running the home is assessed, and the safety of the home's physical fabric and fittings is inspected. Care standards are monitored through inspection visits, of which there must be at least one announced and one unannounced annually. As with the Mental Health Act, a code of practice, *Home Life*, backed up the Act.[5] Home owners can appeal against perceived injustices to a registered homes tribunal, just as psychiatric patients can appeal to a mental health tribunal if they feel they have been unjustly detained. The law on registration and inspection is currently under review. Conservative administrations in the late 1980s and early to mid-1990s wavered between wanting to de-regulate as many services as possible, and realising that registration and inspection are an important safeguard against cowboy operators. It is likely that by the year 2000 all local authority provision will be subject to the same registration standards as private and voluntary homes, and that private home care agencies and small private children's homes looking after fewer than four children will also have to be registered. The trend is to put safety first, which has to be a higher priority than the right to run a business caring for vulnerable people for maximum profit without adequate checks and enforcement of standards. At present, the standards and checks required are far less rigorous than those required for all sorts of consumer goods, which may say something about the low status of residential care.

The registration and inspection of children's homes are covered by the Children Act. As with local authority homes for adults, council children's homes do not have to be registered, although they are inspected. They are supposed to comply with registration standards but whether they do or not varies dramatically up and down the country. Local authority inspectors register and inspect all private children's homes, and government inspectors directly inspect voluntary children's homes such as those run by Barnardo's.

## COMPLAINTS PROCEDURES

Both the Children Act and the NHS and Community Care Act brought in new complaints procedures. The way complaints are handled is a measure of the accountability of an organisation. Historically, social services departments were closed worlds, closed even to the rest of the council they were a part of. Complaints forms intended for young people living in residential units often ended up locked in the desk of the officer in charge. Evidence from retrospective child abuse inquiries suggests that some children in the 1970s and 1980s did tell staff they were being abused, but they were often disbelieved.

These new formal procedures, together with the use of independent investigators and the growing number of whistleblowers who report bad practice either anonymously or to someone trusted within their organisation or to the media on the outside, have all helped to develop greater openness and accountability in social care agencies. A very high proportion of calls received by the organisation, Public Concern at Work, are from social workers. Alison Taylor, a social worker in Clwyd, was sacked after exposing abuse in residential care. She later wrote a stunning fictionalised account of her experience and that of the children.[6] Sue Machin, a senior social worker at Ashworth Special Hospital in Merseyside, was also sacked for speaking out. There are codes of practice for whistleblowing such as the British Association of Social Workers (BASW) code,[7] and internal procedures in many councils, such as a 24-hour independent helpline in Lambeth Council in south London.

While every agency has its own small number of vexatious litigants, unjust complainants who victimise staff with an endless stream of nit-picking grievances and fault-finding, the overwhelming majority of users of social services have low expectations of life and the service they are entitled to, so most incidents that should result in a complaint remain unrecorded and invisible.

The enemies of openness are now as likely to be insurers as staff. Insurers regularly threaten to withdraw cover if any paperwork about an allegation is disclosed to a complainant, even if they have a *prima facie* right of access under access to files legislation. This can make a proper professional response to a complaint, including open communication, hard to maintain.

## OTHER RELEVANT LEGISLATION

The Police and Criminal Evidence Act 1984 sets out the ways in which police interviews should be conducted with children and vulnerable adults. Social workers attend these interviews as 'appropriate adults' to safeguard the rights of those arrested.[8] The Carers (Recognition and Services) Act 1995, implemented April 1996, entitles carers who provide substantial and regular care to someone to an assessment of their own needs as carers. The Direct Payments Act 1996, implemented April 1997, allows local authorities to transfer care budgets directly to a disabled person under 65 to make their own arrangements, such as employing their own carers.

Social services managers also need to be aware of the Race Relations Act 1976, the Sex Discrimination Act 1975, the Disability Discrimination Act 1995 and the Equal Pay Act, in terms of their equal opportunity responsibilities, the requirement on them to ensure ethical work practices, and a host of employment law and regulations such as the Employment Protection (Consolidation) Act 1978, Inland Revenue regulations and European directives which cover staffing issues, such as the regulations for care staff covering the lifting and manual handling of vulnerable people, and the use of safe weight-bearing hoisting equipment. The importance of this is illustrated by industrial tribunal decisions which have gone against local authorities who have tried to substantially reduce or weaken the terms and conditions of, say, home care staff, or who have transferred residential care services to third party organisations. For example, Cornwall County Council transferred their eighteen old people's homes including all their staff to Cornwall Care Ltd. Immediately following the transfer, Cornwall Care Ltd reduced the pay and conditions of the staff transferred, only for this later to be deemed illegal, in a judgement which defeated one of the key purposes of the transfer – saving money. Eventually, the staff were awarded compensation for unfair dismissal, but could not get their old level of salary back.

Staff operating social services legislation have to be aware of the effects of prejudice and oppression on minority groups. Legal decisions about the rights of asylum seekers have confirmed that social services is the safety net of the welfare state, albeit a frayed safety net. Asylum seekers are often trapped in an economic and cultural halfway house. While the entitlement of some to claim housing benefit and income support was withdrawn by the Department of

Social Security in the mid-1990s, judges in the High Court ordered that social services departments had a duty of care which extended to food in the form of vouchers and accommodation. Social workers acting on behalf of disadvantaged groups will often be acting within the law when pressing a particular case or claim, or, for example, when challenging the view of a housing officer that a person claiming to be homeless is a liar.

Some studies have found that discrimination is operating inside social services departments. A report by Iqbal on ethnic minority groups and occupational therapy services found that the average waiting times were 260 days for white service users, 310 days for African Caribbean users and 391 days for Asian users.[9]

Most social services are provided by women care workers for women service users, so gender awareness is crucial. People from ethnic minority communities are over-represented on social services caseloads, so a black perspective is vital. Most users of social services are disadvantaged and lack personal power, perhaps through poverty, victimisation or disability. Social services staff are often accused of being politically correct, and of making decisions based on ideology when a pragmatic approach would be better. Some staff, in pursuit of a vision of society based on greater equality, do undoubtedly build in elements of a personal agenda into care plans, which can then become unduly idealised. However, it is important to realise that some of the common allegations about political correctness refer to child care placement decisions, especially adoption and long-term fostering decisions. The Children Act stipulates that before a child is placed, the racial, religious and cultural background of the child must be taken into account. You would not believe that was the law to listen to some critics! Not to consider these questions risks undermining the psychological development and identity of children in need. Black children, especially African Caribbean children, started to come into care in urban areas in Britain in the late 1960s and 1970s as new immigrant families or mixed-race families broke down under a variety of social pressures. Black children quickly became over-represented in the care system compared with the children of other ethnic groups, and most were placed in residential care in the suburbs or the country, in all-white areas looked after by white houseparents. It was not until the early 1980s that some pioneering family placement projects, like the New Black Families project based in Lambeth, began to recruit foster carers from within black communities. They soon found that recruitment was no more difficult than in any other community, and unearthed considerable community commitment to support black children in need. Their work helped to build a professional momentum which was finally recognised in the Children Act's validation of same-race family placements. Approaching the year 2000, the legal framework for social services, while not as strong as some would wish, is firmly rooted in social justice and equality.

# Chapter 3

# The nuts and bolts of care
## Politics and organisation

Social services departments are part of local government, along with teachers, environmental health officers, street cleaners and planning officers. Including over fifty new authorities from April 1998, created as a result of a local government review and reorganisation of boundaries, there are nearly 200 local authorities in the UK, ranging from enormous counties like Kent and Lancashire and huge conurbations like Birmingham to tiny unitary authorities like Rutland and the Corporation of London. The professional issues facing social services directors in Kent and Rutland are similar, but the management task is a galaxy apart. Indeed, the major local authority areas in the UK contain the largest populations under local authority control in the Western world.

While Whitehall, through the Social Services Inspectorate (formerly the Social Work Service), continues to be responsible for the registration and inspection of voluntary children's homes, secure accommodation provision, and the inspection of local authority social services on a rolling programme, central government has not relished assuming direct responsibility for services which have a low public and political interest or kudos until something goes wrong. Passing responsibility elsewhere is not that easy. For example, the Conservative Government's idea in 1996 to shift responsibility for adoption services away from local authorities to the voluntary sector to punish them for being too politically correct in the way they handled children's placements, presupposed a level of organisation and expertise all over the country which only a new national voluntary sector strategy with a new funding base could have delivered. The incoming Labour Government of 1997 hinted that social services departments might be broken up and directly run from Whitehall through regional community care authorities, similar to health authorities. While an element of this might have been sabre-rattling, it is likely that some of the current artificial boundaries between services will be broken down and realigned within the next decade.

The main government responsibility for social services lies with the Department of Health, through the Secretary of State for Health and a junior minister who carries the social services port-folio. A number of select committees consider health and social services issues. They produced a number of influential reports in the 1980s on the needs of carers, and on the need to rationalise laws relating to children which helped bring about the Children Act. In the 1990s, British social services has been busy trying to implement the massive new policy framework introduced in the early 1990s, which followed extensive campaigning and action for change during the 1970s and 1980s. The relatively low-key end-of-century feel about social services policy-making, apart from high-profile activity on youth crime and managerial reorganisa-tions, is partly explained by it being a time for consolidation, doubtless ahead of a new era of policy-making. Social services has its own stop–go cycle. The search goes on for answers to the big questions. Can youth crime be dramatically reduced? Can child protection and mental health tragedies be avoided? Perhaps even more worrying is the suggestion or hint that intractable social prob-lems might be magically solved.

In the world of social services, the most important civil servants are permanent Department of Health officials and officers in the Social Services Inspectorate, also within the Department of Health. The SSI has a regional structure, and is organised into divisions, the two most important being for policy and inspection. The national SSI programme of inspecting local authority services closely follows policy and legislative changes. From 1996, a new programme of 'joint reviews' of local authority social services departments has been undertaken by the SSI in conjunction with the public spending watchdog, the Audit Commission, in which each local authority's overall performance on social services is being reviewed. The most likely general finding is that while some departments excel in some functions or in providing some specialist services, very few will be found to excel in everything they do. Social services these days is made up of too diverse and complex a group of services to allow for simultaneous excellence. Nevertheless, arising out of the findings of the first joint reviews, it is likely that a tool kit for service improvement, or at least a tool kit for successfully coming through a joint review, can be put together.

The SSI has a liaison arrangement with each social services department through a nominated link inspector. Contact is minimal unless there is a serious problem, and this reflects civil service cutbacks. The onus is placed on local authorities to keep the SSI informed of significant local developments and high-profile cases. While there is a statutory requirement for local authorities to notify the Department of Health of the death of a child in care or on the child protection register, local authorities should supply the SSI with briefing notes on anything out of the ordinary. While this will normally only be logged for intelligence purposes, it is a sound insurance policy. Civil servants themselves work in an uncomfortable buffer zone between suspicious directors of social services and the short-term thinking of ministers who themselves may not be around for long before switching briefs. As professional journeymen, SSI and Department of Health officials have done a lot behind the scenes over the years to safeguard British social services.

How the system operates politically can be illustrated by the backstage process behind the issuing of the White Paper on Social Services two months before the 1997 general election. The Conservative Secretary of State for Health, Stephen Dorrell, wanted to issue a White Paper for a variety of political reasons, some ideological, and others more personal such as his perception that the service delivery system needed a stronger emphasis on achieving value for money, and that inspection and registration services should be placed outside social services departments. Dorrell also had to reflect to a greater or lesser extent the views of Cabinet colleagues, especially the Prime Minister John Major who wanted certain child care services such as adoption moved away from local authorities. Stephen Dorrell had a series of meetings with Sir Herbert Laming and Tom Luce, the two most senior civil servants responsible for British social services.

In those meetings, Laming and Luce, having themselves been thoroughly briefed by civil servants responsible for individual policy areas, indicated to the Secretary of State that his policy objectives could be achieved without wholesale upheaval, in particular that the Children Act had by and large been successfully implemented by local authorities, and that the requirement to involve the private and voluntary sector in providing community care services had also largely been met since the reforms were introduced in 1993. Thus, in time-honoured style, civil servants substantially watered down a politician's strategic ideas into a set of proposals that made sense to the majority of people within the profession. Tom Luce drafted the White Paper, which was then sent back to the Cabinet and the No. 10 Policy Unit for comment and suggested revision. The real tussle had been between professional civil servants and political advisers within the private offices of key Cabinet ministers.

Every local authority has to have a director of social services, or an equivalent nominated senior officer who has responsibility for social services and has the ability to commit resources in response to a particular problem. This requirement is set out in the 1970 Local Authority Social Services Act. While most local authorities in the UK have traditional director posts, some corporate directors are responsible for a number of other departments as well as social services. The more corporate work that directors of social services undertake across councils, the less time they have for social services.

Within local authorities, directors of social services are respon-sible to chief executives, and to elected councillors, in particular the social services committee and the chair of social services who heads that committee. The working relationship between the chief execu-tive and the director of social services needs to be effective and trusting. The same goes for the working relationship between the director of social services and the chair of social services. Ideally they will share similar values, and this is often the key to a successful partnership. If there is a blame culture operating at the top, it will permeate downwards. If the chair gives the director a hard time, blaming him or her for everything that isn't done at the snap of a finger, the director might well do the same with junior staff. Directors of social services these days have to be as political as the politicians, although becoming too closely aligned with any one party can be fatal. A director's basic responsibility is to advise the whole council.

Committees are made up of councillors from parties who are allocated seats according to the prevailing political balance within a council. They meet either during the day or the evening, typically during the day in the counties and in the evening in cities. Social services committees meet between four and six times a year, and consider reports prepared by officers on policy and financial matters. The reports will usually have been planned in consultation between leading councillors and the director. The director and the chair of social services will usually aim to achieve a cross-party consensus. Unless the relationships between different political groups on a council are particularly hostile, social services committees are usually one of the least politicised committees, where councillors reach agreements relatively easily, apart from decisions on cuts packages! However, no two groups of councillors are the same. Councillors in one authority can be fairly laid back and easy going, allowing the managers they appoint high levels of discretion, while in other authorities they can be highly involved in all aspects of detailed operational work, sometimes destructively. The norm is somewhere in the middle.

## HOW SOCIAL SERVICES DEPARTMENTS WORK DAY TO DAY

Since the early 1990s, virtually every social services department in the UK has been organised into specialist teams. Generic teams of the 1970s and 1980s, who dealt with every referral, but tended to be embroiled in children's cases at the expense of all adult services, have been consigned to social work history. By the late 1990s the only truly generic social services staff left are emergency duty staff, who cover every service outside normal working hours, and directors of social services, who themselves may not be social workers. Remote parts of the UK such as the Western Isles of Scotland and the Scilly Isles do retain a small number of generic staff covering a group of islands, supplemented by island-based services such as home care into which other services like a meals-on-wheels service are integrated.

Following corporate reorganisations, some authorities like the new Milton Keynes unitary authority have abolished social services departments altogether, integrating children's services with education services, and community care services with housing services. Some new unitary authorities, through being small and local, may bring services closer to the public than a large anonymous county could ever do. One authority, Dumfries and Galloway in Scotland, has begun to integrate social services with its local health service, seeking to form a single health and social care service similar to Northern Ireland health and social services boards. Just as some authorities like Islington and Tower Hamlets pursued radical decentralisation policies in the 1980s, experimental structures in the late 1990s bring both excitement and confusion in their wake. There is no evidence that one structure works better than another. Each has its champion. Indeed, some new structures abolish old arrangements only for those same old arrangements to be revived in future years by new leaders in yet another set of changes which in turn are touted as unavoidable. Restructurings produce no discernible service benefits unless other changes are made at the same time, such as changes in the values and culture of the organisation. Employee involvement is a vital but often missing component of change programmes.[1] The impact of change on service users is rarely considered.

Directors of social services work at the professional, political and managerial level. In their work, they have to interpret and reflect social political and legal trends in matters as wide ranging as teenage drinking, pre-teen pregnancies, voluntary euthanasia sought by people with extremely painful degenerative illnesses, and what to tell the public about paedophiles, in addition to steering their organisations through a minefield of legal and bureaucratic complexity. They are involved with a range of people in central government, through professional associations like the Association of Directors of Social Services and through Local Government Associations, which are the umbrella groups for local councils in England and Wales, and through regional political forums like the Association for London Government. Further down the management chain, social work managers work strategically and operationally in respect of day-to-day services.

Social services staff tend to work in small teams run by a team leader or a team manager. Teams vary from four to five up to fifteen to twenty in size, the ideal number being six to eight. Smaller teams increase management costs and overheads, so the trend is towards larger teams made up of more than one professional group. The most effective teams share a workload, maximise internal cover and minimise differences. As Terry Bamford puts it:

> There is a strong participative culture within social work. It is, and remains, one of the great strengths of social services organisations. Long before management gurus were stressing the vital role of communication, involvement and job enrichment, social services were practising it.[2]

It is usually best if staff teams are mixed in terms of age, race and gender, because this reflects the variety of local populations. Teams need a mix of experienced and new staff, and great care has to be taken to avoid the recruitment of a totally inexperienced team without old heads around to put things into perspective.

## INDEPENDENT SOCIAL WORKERS

Social workers or managers work independently or freelance for four main reasons. The flexibility suits some, especially if they're at the 'in-between' stage in their own lives or careers. Others have no choice because they've been made redundant. The freedom from being managed, and from the usual organisational ups and downs, is attractive to some. A fourth group think that new legislation and systems have down-graded the status of social workers and professional staff. Working independently, some feel, allows them to work to a higher professional standard than they can inside a local authority. However, most independent social workers depend on public agencies for work. There are few privately funded social workers, so the criticism of nursing and medical staff in NHS hospitals which goes something like 'they'd be nice to you if you were a private patient' is one criticism that can't be made of too many social workers!

For management, it is tempting to reduce the number of full-time staff and replace them with independent staff working either on an hourly basis or on a price for each piece of work. Inspection or registration reports are an example where employing freelance inspectors is substantially cheaper than using in-house staff. Guardian *ad litem* services are another. On the other hand, independent social workers can veer off at a tangent and sometimes find it hard to work within an organisation's overall objectives. They also offer little continuity from one job to the next. If it adopts a commissioning-only structure, an organisation can lose its culture and values which really need to be maintained by groups of permanent staff working together over a period of time delivering front-line services.

## SOCIAL SERVICES IN RURAL AREAS

The Rural Development Commission defines a rural area as one where communities comprise fewer than 10,000 people, which means 20 per cent of the UK population. Social work in rural areas is primarily characterised by the physical distances involved. Social workers can travel up to 50 miles in some parts of the country to make a single visit. Distance also increases the isolation of vulnerable people. A strong local voluntary sector is vital, including local branches of national voluntary organisations like the Women's Royal Voluntary Service (WRVS), so that at the village level there is a support network in place, involving local GPs and volunteers backed up by other professionals outside the immediate geographical area.

Rural services depend upon fast and clear communication but, then, so do services next door to each other in the inner city. Small groups of volunteers in four Bedfordshire villages carry pagers which can be called at any time of the day or night by residents in trouble. Home-from-hospital schemes run by the Red Cross ensure older people discharged from hospital immediately receive friendship and practical support. WRVS volunteers deliver hot meals to housebound people in many parts of the country. In north Herefordshire, a mobile day centre, consisting of two minibuses and a 16-foot trailer, tours village halls offering chiropody services, health checks and hairdressing.

## HOW SOCIAL SERVICES IS FINANCED

Social services are in the top ten UK public spending programmes, spending over £8 billion a year at 1997–8 prices. One-third of the overall budget is spent on residential care. One-tenth is spent on each of the following: day care services, social workers, home care services and the administration of social services including management. The remaining 30 per cent goes on relatively small services such as foster care and voluntary sector contracts.

Since 1993, local authorities have been expected to raise as much of their budget as possible through charging, and this, plus other financial pressures, has led most social services departments to charge older people and disabled people for a proportion of the cost of their care packages. Any charge levied must be reasonable and must take into account ability to pay. About 13 per cent of total expenditure is recovered from charging for services, especially adult residential services. The dangers of excessive charging are that people will decline to use the service, which is all right if there are alternatives, but not if the service user as a result becomes more vulnerable. All authorities waive charges in certain cases, or do not enforce the charge if there is no realistic likelihood of collection.

The bottom line is that a service must be provided even if a debt is incurred.

While there was great opposition to the introduction of charging when it was first mooted, most authorities have now accepted they have no choice if they are to maintain service levels. Disability groups fiercely lobby against local authorities who take back most of their disability-related benefits such as the care component of Disability Living Allowances, arguing that higher benefits are needed to pay for a higher cost of living, because disabled people often have to pay more for basic goods and services such as extra transport and heating.

Capital expenditure on social services is low which reflects both the restrictions on local authority capital spending and policy shifts away from residential care to care in the community, in the shape of foster care for children and intensive home care for adults. Some new capital schemes are being financed under the Private Finance Initiative, through which private sector investment is used for public sector building or repairs programmes.

Social services are funded through the Revenue Support Grant, which is paid annually in a single block grant to each local authority to run all its services. Government indicates to local authorities what it thinks it should spend on each service, in the form of a Standard Spending Assessment (SSA). For social services, there is an overall SSA, and within that a children's services SSA, an elderly services SSA, and an 'other' SSA which covers disability services. Local authorities do not have to allocate resources internally to SSA levels, as these are for guidance only, and the underlying methodology for calculating SSAs has been repeatedly questioned. SSAs are calculated using a range of general population data. They are prone to miss key local trends and variations that do not necessarily show up in broad demographic profiles. At worst, the SSA is a virtual budget. Some social services departments spend 50 per cent above it, others up to 40 per cent below, but despite intense protest from individual local authorities and their associations, it has emerged unscathed as a formula in recent years. The same protests about the unfairness of the resource allocation mechanism are voiced in health authorities in relation to the capitation funding formula.

As with all other council departments, social services officers and councillors determine annually by how much the social services budget goes up or down. For the last few years, the settlement for local government, announced annually in the Chancellor's budget at the end of November, has been poor, necessitating annual reductions in expenditure. Few social services departments were able to avoid making large and damaging cuts in the late 1980s and this trend has intensified in the 1990s. For many authorities, cuts in the mid-1990s have been the most root and branch of all. Increases in demand at the same time as reductions in budgets drive down service levels and standards. Given the macro-economic indicators for public sector borrowing and expenditure, it is unlikely the trend will be reversed over the next five to ten years. As the cuts deepen, so the political debate about welfare hots up. Social services budgets are cash-limited, which means demand has to be regulated between competing needs. One reason the government cash-limits welfare budgets is that if all expenditure was underwritten, it thinks local authorities would have no incentive to make efficiency savings. In many parts of the country, budgets are so limited that a new residential or nursing home placement can only be made if someone else who is being financially supported dies, thus releasing a new 'person worth' of funding. The Labour Government removed the Conservatives' capping limits on local authorities' own local tax-raising powers, so that local residents will be able to decide whether to pay more for their local education service and for local social services. Whether residents in many parts of the country would vote extra cash out of their own pockets for social services is a moot question. The government will however retain powers to keep councils in line financially.

Additional funding is made available to social services departments through annual one-off specific grants, like the AIDS support grant (ASG), and the Drugs and Alcohol Specific Grant (DASG). These specific grants are gradually being phased out, which will inevitably lead to reductions in services as some local authorities will not be able to pick up all of the funding. This will hurt the voluntary sector most as contracting with the voluntary sector is a precondition for some grants.

Since April 1993, the government has provided additional resources to local authorities to take over the responsibility for all new placements of adults in residential care who before then were funded directly by the social security system. A Special Transitional Grant (STG) was calculated for each local authority, and paid annually. It is due to end in March 1999. Before April 1993 the social security budget for these placements was spiralling out of

control. Many local authorities transferred their residential establishments to what Lesley Hoyes refers to as 'non-public
management in order to pass the costs on to the apparently open-
ended social security budget'.[3] The major loopholes by which this
could be done were quickly closed by the government. Since then,
the budget has been cash-limited to local authorities and it is no
surprise that they have found it difficult to stay within their allocated budget. A cynic might say this was the main reason for the
transfer of responsibility from central to local government in the
first place. Long-term funding shortfalls remain a serious problem.
Unlike the health service, which can be transformed in part through
technological improvements, social services are labour-intensive.
Quick fixes usually turn out to be botches.

The local authority financial year runs from one April to the next.
Many local authorities have devolved their budgets down to front-
line teams and establishments, so that local managers can use their
part of the budget flexibly to support people with the greatest needs
in their part of the service. Devolution can eliminate the inherent
delays and administration costs in constantly referring expenditure
proposals up the hierarchy, as long as local managers know the rules
about what can and cannot be spent, and as long as they are supplied
with an accurate financial information monitoring system.

The main difficulty in operating a devolved budget is the sheer
number of spending pressures, particularly from the budgets used to
purchase care services. By definition these are volatile and unpre-
dictable. For instance, in Essex in 1996 twenty-four foster carers, paid
at local authority rates, decided to break away and join an independent fostering agency. The county council felt they could not move
the children, and therefore at a stroke had to pay an extra half a
million pounds as the same placements suddenly cost double.
Because of these vagaries, underspent budgets get raided to cover
overspending elsewhere, which in turn can lead to prudent managers
becoming demoralised because all their hard work fails to lead to a
reinvestment in their own service but is used to bail out other services
that they suspect, often unfairly, are run by spendthrifts.

Ideally, social services should be decentralised to the local level,
so that local people are at least aware of their local social services
office. However, local offices are expensive to run, so site rationali-
sations are taking place, with staff tending to operate from central
bases. In the health service, acute hospitals have closed through staff
and skill shortages, so that where acute hospitals remain open, they

have the range of skills to provide high quality 24-hour emergency care for all medical conditions, through a so-called 'critical professional mass'. The same holds for social services.

## STAFF IN SOCIAL SERVICES

Looking after others is not what it used to be. There are no easy service users any more. Children in residential care can be violent and challenging, threatening staff, wrecking property and injuring themselves. Over half of the residents in a local authority old people's home might be suffering from dementia. Home care staff have to rush from one personal care job to another, in order to fit in extra demands. They often have to be taken off their own lower-priority work to cover someone else's higher-priority cases, thus breaking the bond they have gradually built up with users, and often with carers. The pace of change in its own right undermines standards of care, making everyone involved more anxious and stressed. Residents in a group home for mentally ill people might assault staff sexually and physically on occasions. Another resident with a severe brain injury might lash out at random through sheer frustration. Social services look after the people no-one else will, so when there are violent and destructive incidents, staff have to carry on as best they can because there are rarely any viable alternative placements. Often their only defence is to threaten to refuse to carry on caring, which would be a violation of the duty of care and leads mostly to tense brinkmanship with service users, with managers, and with other agencies about who should be taking responsibility.

Child protection social workers are called upon to make hairline decisions about whether a child is safe at home or not. They have to do this without having a legal power of entry into people's homes, unless there is compelling *prima facie* evidence a child is in immediate danger. Social workers have to rely upon establishing a relationship with the family in order to carry out basic child protection work. Social workers in community mental health teams wonder if the person they haven't been able to contact might kill himself or someone else. Is he in but not opening the door? Shall we break the door down? In family proceedings courts, child care social workers are often relentlessly criticised by a posse of lawyers representing all sides of a family in a contested case, where the family are captive clients, there but not wanting to be there, angry, with their backs up against the wall. This perpetual attrition may be one reason for the difficulties most local authorities have experienced in recruiting social workers. Many authorities have vacancy levels as high as 30 per cent. Some authorities have had to go abroad to find staff. In 1996, Essex recruited twenty-seven social workers following a recruitment campaign in Canada.

Stress and sickness levels amongst social services staff are high for an occupational group. An area manager in Northumberland social services, John Walker, successfully sued Northumberland County Council for £200,000, on the basis that he was placed back in the same stressful job after a period of sick leave for stress, and after he warned his employer he could no longer cope. At its most extreme, burn-out can lead staff to withdraw psychologically and emotionally from work, leading to service users being neglected.

Social workers have to be able to cope with seeing people go through great pain or trauma. They have to 'get next to them' in order to understand the nature of their problems and help them see if a way through can be found. Most of us go through life with the minimum of trauma, especially those of us who have not been caught up in a war or an episode of random acute violence. We hear or read about other people's experiences rather than have them for ourselves. For most of us, the most extreme images come from television sets or the newspapers, whereas for most social workers, even those who are young and straight out of college, the shocking extremes of human behaviour present themselves daily, live. One of the authors, while on emergency duty, was called to a flat because children could be heard crying. When he let himself in using a neighbour's key, he saw a 3 year old and a 5 year old huddled together looking at their mother, who had been strangled and was dead on the floor, and their father, who had hung himself from the curtain rail. The children looked bewildered and petrified. Images like that burn themselves into social workers' minds and remain there for the rest of their lives.

So why do people work in social services? Such a personal job implies personal reasons. These can include having grown up in a caring role within your own family and pursuing that as a way of life; having had similar experiences yourself such as being in care and being drawn towards the same system you had a connection with; or simply wanting to help people, arising out of a strong sense of anger at the way vulnerable people are treated. It is fashionable to deny altruism, and claim that everyone going into social work has to have an ulterior or even a sinister motive. That underestimates the genuine desire of young people wanting to go into a profession like social work to 'make a difference'. Mature older people also feel that having lived their life in a certain way, possibly somewhat selfishly, they now want to put something back in, either professionally or as a volunteer.

Social workers are a diverse bunch, but they rarely conform to some of the wilder stereotypes the public are fond of like neo-hippies, sociology-obsessed political activists or religious extremists. The few who use so-called politically correct language tend to be middle class and confined to the London area. Generally, social workers are like any other work group. Some get together on a personal basis, but then statistically over 60 per cent of personal relationships start at work so this is hardly surprising. In the days before social services became more regimented, a male social worker known to one of the authors confronted a father who abused his children by pinning him up against a wall and threatening to beat him up if he did it again. Fortunately, that kind of do-it-yourself social work has all but disappeared, just like the friendly local 'bobby' who gave wayward children a 'clip round the ear'.

Most social services staff today are indistinguishable from staff in any other profession, at least in looks and dress. Surveys of the readership of *Community Care* magazine suggest that politically over 65 per cent of social workers support the Labour Party.[4] Nearly 50 per cent of staff in social services are members of the public sector trade union, Unison. Generally, industrial relations in social services in the 1990s, like everywhere else in the UK, have been quiet apart from occasional flashpoints. It wasn't always so. There were bitter disputes in many social services departments in the 1970s and 1980s. Some disputes resulted in long strikes which took half a decade to recover from. Most social services staff enjoy their job, against the odds, and maintain a positive optimistic outlook. They are not especially good at explaining what they do, or at cultivating a robust public image, and their professional associations, like the British Association of Social Workers, and institutions, like the National Institute for Social Work, are unable to gain sustained media coverage outside the professional press. Positive developments are under-reported. Scandals are sensationalised. If you work in social services, a single mistake may be more significant in career terms than 1,000 well-handled incidents. No professional group could remain entirely optimistic in those circumstances. Medical negligence, for example, is much better hidden from public scrutiny.

Overall, social services staff are a kind of professional Eurosceptic – their natural instinct is to be suspicious and they rarely combine forces with neighbouring authorities even when a better and cheaper set of services might be provided by collaborating. There is a hierarchy of suspicion. Local residents are suspicious of users of social services, users of social services are suspicious of social services staff, and social services departments tend to be suspicious and paranoid about the world outside. Having said that, things would be far worse if social services provision was taken away from local government, where it at least has some checks and balances, to establish a free-standing national organisation. Such a body would end up being the most secretive of all quangos, a sort of MI5 of the care world.

In fact, social workers represent only 12 per cent of the 350,000 social services staff in local authorities, and twice this number of staff work in the independent sector, the majority of whom are care staff such as home carers and residential staff. Altogether, a million people are employed in UK social services, one in twenty of the working population, the vast majority of them unqualified. There is an increasing casualisation of the social services workforce, with fewer permanent staff and more sessional staff and use of short-term contracts. Full-time care staff are increasingly employed on a more flexible contractual basis, whereby they receive no extra payments for evening, night or weekend working, but simply have to work the hours their employer needs them. Staff need planning for. Without workforce planning co-ordinated nationally or at least regionally, the right skill mix of staff will not be available in future. In Hertfordshire in 1997, there were serious shortages of nurses in nursing homes and home care workers in private home care agencies. This growing national problem is compounded by the considerable number of women in their fifties who are suffering from weak and sometimes damaged backs and knees as a result of over twenty years of caring. Thousands more home care workers will be needed nationally over the next ten years, but little effort is being made nationally to identify and train such a workforce. The key relationship in workforce planning is the one between the workforce and the service user profile. Basically, staff have to be right for the people who need help. There has to be a fit of skills, attitudes and values. The same applies to the agencies with whom a social services department contracts or sub-contracts. Staff in those agencies also need to fit the user profile in an area.

Tucked away in the remote corners of social services departments are other groups of staff who rarely hit the headlines, such as welfare rights workers who advocate for individual service users with the Benefits Agency. They also liaise with Benefits Agency managers which can be an important local contribution to anti-poverty work, limiting as far as possible benefit officers' over-harsh interpretation of their own regulations. Take-up campaigns about underclaimed benefits can lead to gains in income for poor people of hundreds of thousands of pounds annually in a local area. Many people either don't know what they're entitled to, or else the application forms are too daunting to complete. Welfare rights staff have also helped to establish local credit unions, as a form of community banking in which people too poor to be given credit cards can at least borrow small sums on a low interest basis rather than being exploited by local money-lenders or pawnbrokers.

Other staff, usually administrators, arrange for property to be secured and an estate wound up if someone dies without resources and without having any relatives or friends to sort things out. Social services also have a duty to take pets into care either after death as part of the Protection of Property responsibility, or in other cases if someone goes into residential care in an emergency. A social worker known to one of the authors went to take an inventory of a flat and secure it, only to be met by a huge boa constrictor curled up on the sofa. This was in the middle of London!

Staff with relatively little status in organisations, such as receptionists, hold great power and sway with service users. A hostile receptionist can subtly force a person needing help to give up and leave an office before the story they need to offload is told. The importance of attitude can be expressed by thinking of social care agencies as personality-intensive as well as labour-intensive. Communication skills and positive attitudes are vital attributes for staff at all levels.

The Labour Government intends to establish a new professional body to regulate social services staff in the same way that nurses, doctors and architects are. Such a General Social Care Council would focus on conduct and professional standards, and be a safeguard against the small minority of social services staff who abuse service users or who are guilty of other types of professional malpractice. Registration with such a statutory body could act as a passport for professional staff, deregistration having the opposite effect. To be effective against wily paedophiles, or slick fraudsters, a register or council would need to have more teeth than existing professional bodies, or the current central government registers like the Department of Health consultancy list and the Department for Education and Employment's List 99, on which staff convicted of offences against children can be placed for prospective employers to run recruitment checks against it. These lists are neither up to date nor comprehensive. Lists themselves are dangerous. They give the illusion of protection, whereas sinister operators find their way into new jobs even when they have been sacked from their last job and their name has been entered on every possible list. Sometimes this is because personnel staff inside employing organisations attach insufficient significance to information in an applicant's background. In one local authority in 1995, a personnel manager took the view that a criminal conviction in the 1970s for streaking down the high street of a seaside town should not affect the appointment of a supply teacher in local schools. The offence had not been declared by the applicant and had only come to light after a statutory police check. The teacher went on to abuse a number of children.

Standards of public service have only received a high level of attention since MPs were involved in numerous high-profile scandals, resulting in the Nolan Committee being established. Social workers are protected from too challenging a definition of proper conduct by being local authority employees, which sets a common standard for refuse collectors and birth and death registrars as well as social services staff.

Complaints about social services staff suggest attitude and behaviour are as much a problem as lack of resources or delay in putting in a service. Complainants talk of an arrogant or patronising attitude. Despite the trendy rhetoric about user involvement and a customer-facing ethos, social services departments still need to gain public confidence by being more open in their day-to-day work. As social work has never quite achieved the status of an acknowledged profession in the UK, with the lingering implication that what social services staff do is merely glorified common sense, staff may feel they have to publicise what they do. A service user in a day centre visited by one of the authors put it well when he said, 'The staff here give you a nice feeling. They look after you. There's a happy smile on their faces. They're pleased to see you when you come here.' But behind those smiles will surely have been clear positive leadership, skilled management at the centre, and a well-motivated staff group who excel at teamwork.

## SUPERVISION OF STAFF

In supervision sessions or meetings, managers sit down with staff to discuss cases, especially the content of assessments and care plans. Supervision is a vital teaching and training tool as newly qualified social workers are often allocated complex cases they feel ill-prepared for. The most experienced social workers often go into management, leaving the most inexperienced staff to deal with difficult and complex direct work. Supervision helps to bridge the gaps.

Supervision is a good way of identifying staff under stress, and of planning with them how to recover confidence in their work. Social workers regularly encounter highly distressing situations. Supervision can be a safe haven to share experiences and come to terms with them. Physical and verbal abuse of social services staff is unfortunately common. A survey carried out by *Community Care* magazine found that twice as many social workers were assaulted as police officers in the Metropolitan Police area.[5] Social workers can sometimes find themselves in the homes of extremely violent people without realising it, because the referral information has not been collated properly, or because of the nature of the situation, such as the need to remove a child from a parent. While only a small number of social workers have been killed in the line of duty, at least one was stalked before being killed (Isabel Schwarz, a hospital social worker who was killed by Sharon Campbell, a psychiatric patient, at Bexley Hospital in 1982), and social workers have been taken hostage. Verbal abuse is far more common, and to some extent social workers get used to it. Nevertheless, it can destroy confidence and the steadfastness needed to think clearly and act confidently in conflict situations. Staff who are assaulted should always be offered special leave, counselling and access to legal advice.

Supervision in residential and day care settings is the forum for discussing how to cope with particular residents or groups of residents, and looks at how effectively staff are working 'on the floor'. Supervision has a long history in social work, and is the main quality control measure of front-line work. Supervision used to be more reflective, but pressures are such nowadays that what should be an uninterrupted activity can easily be disrupted by the need to deal with an emergency, or by either the supervisor or the supervisee feeling distracted by other pressures. Supervision levels have undoubtedly been reduced since managers themselves have been allocated ever-wider spans of responsibility. Greater workloads, especially the volume of assessments, mean that identifying the right subject to focus on in supervision is like throwing a treble twenty in darts when the dartboard is spinning round. With hindsight, when cases go wrong, it is obvious that a particular case merited greater discussion and a change of plan earlier, but at the time that case could have been indistinguishable from many others.

## SOCIAL WORK METHODS

After brief encounters with psychoanalysis and attachment theory in the 1960s, community development, radical social work and group work in the 1970s, and family therapy and systems theory in the 1980s, individual casework is now the mainstream social work method, although at least one study found social workers made use of over eighty different theories, which suggests confusion as well as eclecticism.[6]

Social work has an impressive track record of developing new ways of working. Use of a life-story book, which is an organised photographic and literary record of a child in care's life, or indeed an older person's life looking back in old age, has been a valued and original tool now in regular use in a number of professional settings outside social work.

The most popular social work methods today are counselling and task-centred work, probably because they fit in best with modern service requirements to bring about defined and measurable change in someone's life in the shortest possible time. All social work methods, such as cognitive behavioural therapy, personal construct therapy and task-centred short-term work, have a potential application in the right situation, and the competent practitioner is able to use a range of methods to suit the occasion.

Whatever method is adopted, all social services staff must have a basic understanding of human nature. They must be able to understand how people tick, and be aware of the impact of critical life events such as bereavement and the process of mourning, relationship breakdown and the associated anger and loss, and virtually all other social and personal life events which bring people to them either voluntarily or compulsorily.

Sheer pressure of work has had a major impact on social work methods. Today is not the time to be brave. New legislation and higher public expectations are demanding a standards-based framework for services to individuals which only a focused specialist casework service can ensure. Innovative projects are still being developed up and down the country and always will be, but the majority of authorities cannot afford to invest in the development time and expense needed to build up large-scale alternatives to casework. Other smaller-scale approaches include group treatment programmes, for example with sex offenders or with people dependent on drugs or alcohol; team-held work in which a proportion of cases are held collectively by team members, any of whom can respond; and small-group support, where groups such as carers are supported through regular meetings and funding for self-help.

Within the casework umbrella, the current emphasis on measuring outcomes means that social work, like health treatments, will have to become evidence-based. New centres like the Centre for Evidence-Based Social Services at Exeter University will be influential in linking research and practice to outcomes. Health policy has a head start in measuring outcomes. For example, new cancer treatments have been clearly linked to lower mortality rates. Finding the right ways of measuring success in social services, using more sophisticated measurements than numbers of people seen and other crude input data, will be needed to prove the service is worthy of higher levels of public funding. Part of this proof may lie in being more positive about social work within the service itself. Being surrounded by so much doom and gloom, both on the institutional side and in the lives of users, can lead to an overstated pessimism. Many new services, such as community mental health teams, are acts of faith, but they are likely to lead to better outcomes in mental health than leaving people on long-stay hospital wards. A positive and upbeat belief in what is being done is a precondition of it becoming excellent.

# Chapter 4

# For the child's sake
## Services for children

A century ago, children formed 30 per cent of the UK population. Now it's 20 per cent. The UK has the highest proportion of single-parent families in the European Union. Half of absent parents lose touch with their children completely, and half of the rest see their children less than once a month.[1] In terms of social trends, children smoke more, go to church less, have more disposable income, take more drugs, commit fewer crimes and travel more. More children than ever before go on to higher education.[2] On the other hand, a small number of serious violent crimes, including rape and murder, committed by young people against other young people or adults, often in gangs, suggests that some young people living in urban areas are stacking up high levels of anger, resentment and lawlessness at a young age and see few personal opportunities ahead. They carry knives and replica guns as fashion accessories. Situational crime born out of bravado is rife.

Events and social issues which preoccupy us today will be of little concern to the next generation. In 1985, Barnet Council took legal proceedings to make Baby 'C', born to a surrogate mother, a Ward of Court. The case was eventually lost and relatively little has been heard about surrogacy since, partly because adverse publicity forces such practices underground. It may be that twenty-five years from now, social workers specialising in frontier biology will take the first parentless cloned baby into care. In twenty-five years' time, there will be about the same number of children as now, but the average age for a woman to give birth to her first child will have gone up to 28. Young people in Spain and Italy now leave home on average at the same age – 28. It is likely the trend in the UK will drift in that direction.

Perceptions of risk also change over time. Thirty years ago, if a

14-year-old girl became pregnant, the odds on her baby coming into care were high. Today, this hardly ever happens. The girl and probably her own mother would be given considerable support to look after the child, and educational provision would be made available so the girl's schooling need not suffer unduly.

Social services for children has always been dominated by two policy objectives. One is to make sure children are cared for properly. The other is to control the children no-one else can. The problem with the first is that near-certainty of danger is needed before you can intervene in family life, and even when it has, social services has not been able to care for children all that well or safely itself. The catalogue of abuse children in care have suffered is testimony to that. The problem with the second is that there is no easy way to control children, or adults for that matter, who are out of control. A more limited secondary objective has arisen: to make sure children behave within tolerable limits without being able to do much about the underlying reasons they are out of control in the first place. This reflects badly on national policy, as destructive or self-destructive children frequently grow up to be destructive or self-destructive adults. It is a very limited policy objective that does not tackle root causes. This does not detract from the much greater number of people who benefit from good relationships with professionals as children and grow up to be adults without any problems, or indeed who grow up in care and go on to be famous, like Bruce Oldfield, the fashion designer.

## CHILD PROTECTION

Some parents dislike or even hate their children. Hard though it is to accept, some parents are permanently angry with their children, seeing them as the cause of all their problems. Rejected children can face life-long anxiety and depression as a result. This is just one small point on the spectrum of child abuse, which stretches all the way from long-running undermining of a child's self-esteem to horrific sexual and physical attacks including torture and murder. Child abuse is not random. A high percentage of child abusers have been abused themselves as children. Child abuse is not new. Gender-based infanticide, organised sexual abuse and unchallenged cruelty are part of the history of childhood across cultures. In many Third World countries today, children live on the street, eking out a living by selling matches, chewing gum, flowers, as 'teeny-mafia' minders of parking bays for motorists, or as child labour where that is the economic reality.

Child protection work is the most visible social work of all, because of public interest. Social workers investigate all referrals that suggest a child is being abused. Very few anonymous calls about child abuse are malicious, so each child and family must be visited and assessed before a conclusion can be reached that there is nothing to worry about. All referrals are discussed between social services and the police, as child abuse is a crime. Evidence of abuse is notoriously hard to gather. A lot of information is too impressionistic to be acted upon. *In extremis*, a social services department in conjunction with the police, whose resources usually won't stretch to covert surveillance methods, might hire a private investigator to undertake covert operations such as using concealed cameras to find out what is happening to a child at serious risk. The general public would be surprised at the lengths some departments will go when they are concerned about the well-being of a particular child. Child protection procedures are organised through local area child protection committees (ACPCs), and a copy of local procedures can be seen in schools and libraries. ACPCs are statutory bodies, made up of senior representatives of local child protection agencies like social services, health, the police and education. Each local ACPC in the country must submit an annual report to the Department of Health covering the work it is doing each year to prevent child abuse in its community.

Trends in child abuse are difficult to pinpoint. While more cases of sexual abuse were reported in the mid-1980s to mid-1990s than in earlier decades, this may be due to an increased awareness of a form of abuse which has been with us for centuries, rather than an increase in underlying levels. An explosion of reporting also accompanies any new discovery, which gets hyped out of all proportion until it settles down. As global cultures start to merge because of sustained emigration and changes in national boundaries, so social workers have to be aware of cultural differences in seeking to understand and define what constitutes child abuse.

Rare blood disorders which cause external skin changes in African and Chinese children have been mistakenly diagnosed as physical abuse. Russian peasants calm their baby boys by sucking their penises, but it would be wrong to automatically label this as child abuse. Many parents from non-UK cultures sleep with their children until the children are almost teenagers, and this should not be defined as unsavoury or unsafe. A Turkish paediatrician told one of the authors that he found the British practice of putting children to sleep in separate rooms at a young age quite barbaric! On the other hand, cultural practices like female circumcision have been condemned by women's groups all over the world as sadistic and unjustifiable. Social workers in the UK have to apply a flexible definition of child abuse, which respects cultural differences but which seeks to protect children from real danger, whatever their culture.

In 1994, there were 160,000 referrals to social services departments suggesting a child might be at risk: 120,000 of these (75 per cent) resulted in home visits. No further action was taken in 80,000 cases. Investigations in 40,000 cases led to a child protection conference being convened: 24,000 children were placed on child protection registers. Ninety-five per cent of children referred to child protection services remained at home. Of the other 5 per cent, most were soon re-united with their families.[3]

In 1995, 35,000 children in the UK were on local child protection registers, which are lists of children at high levels of risk of being harmed by a parent or carer, almost always in their own home. Considering 24,000 children were placed on such registers in 1994, this shows that children come onto and move off local registers with great frequency. Children are registered following a decision of a case conference, which is a meeting involving professional staff from different organisations, like head teachers, police officers and social workers. Parents and older children should attend these conferences, but attendance levels vary considerably across the country. Once registered, the conference reconvenes at least every six months until a view is formed that the child is no longer in danger. At that point, the child's name is removed from the register and involvement with the family usually comes to an end. The system tends to register children after abuse has taken place, the value of which has to be questioned. The routine removal of children if nothing serious happens for 1–2 years also belies the long-term nature of less visible and dramatic abuse that children suffer. It would be better to have much smaller registers triggered by much higher levels of concern than the current catch-all threshold, and to then put a multi-agency care plan in place for children over a much longer period of time. Whether or not a child's name is entered on a register also varies with geography. Between 1995 and 1997, register numbers dropped by 25 per cent in a sample of twenty-one authorities, and rose by 47 per cent in one and 25 per cent in another five.[4] These inexplicable fluctuations are unfair, both in whom they protect and whom they stigmatise.

Child abuse cases now show a roughly equal split between physical abuse, sexual abuse, chronic neglect and prolonged and destructive emotional abuse. Some less frequent types of abuse are random abuse by individual strangers and abuse within paedophile rings. While abuse from paedophiles represents a relatively small element of child abuse statistics overall, cases arouse great public concern. The concern is valid, as paedophiles systematically prey upon vulnerable isolated children, as well as sometimes opportunistically abducting children. Most children who disappear in this way are never seen again. A small number are whisked abroad to be used in child pornographic films and other paedophile activities. Many end up working in the sex industry as adults.

There is much talk within the social work profession about 'refocusing' children's services to be more supportive of families, and for social workers to be less intrusive. This follows a general realisation that between 1975 and 1995, services to children and families concentrated too much on assessment and investigation, and too little on helping families. However, care has to be taken that managers and practitioners do not avoid difficult child protection decisions and promote a family support approach simply because it involves less conflict. The families who pose the most threat to children are often the hardest to investigate and the most reluctant to accept help, however sweetened the pill.

Caution is essential. The failure to protect a vulnerable child strikes at the very heart of public confidence in social services. Between 1975 and 1995, several children in Britain were killed by their parents or the live-in partner of a parent, after social services departments had been made aware of possible risks to the child yet under-estimated them. The social services roll call of shame is a depressing one. Jasmine Beckford,[5] Maria Colwell,[6] Tyra Henry,[7] Kimberley Carlile[8] – each death and many more led to separate independent inquiries, the recommendations of which overlapped. The messages from inquiries did not seem to get through to staff on the ground, although the fear of making a mistake undoubtedly did.

In the late 1980s, when public confidence was at its lowest, the phenomenon of over-reaction was the next to be highlighted. In Cleveland, in 1987, social services took over 100 children into care as a result of what was virtually a mass diagnosis of sexual abuse. Using a controversial method of forensic analysis called 'reflex anal dilatation' (RAD) as evidence of buggery, paediatricians alerted social services and the police to what they thought was a discovery of sexual abuse in children who came to their clinics of near epidemic proportions. Medical evidence was split about whether RAD could only be caused by sexual abuse, or whether there were other possible physiological explanations. Most children were returned to their parents following High Court decisions in their favour, because of a lack of corroborative proof that the alleged abuses took place.[9]

This does not mean most of those children were not abused, merely that there was insufficient proof to make a series of irreversible decisions to remove children from their parents for good. In the same way that abuse in care sometimes follows on from abuse at home, so the trauma of abuse for some children is followed by the trauma of having to give evidence against their alleged abuser in court (see Chapter 12 for a case study of the impact of a court process on both children, parents and professionals). Child witness support projects have been able to reduce this anxiety for children, and in some parts of the country the legal process is deliberately speeded up in recognition of the distress caused to child witnesses by excessive delay. The legacy of Cleveland in the history of social services is unclear. The diagnoses were made in good faith, even though there may have been an element of finding what you wanted to find. Even then, efforts to save children from years of painful abuse were well intentioned. Social workers are now more socialised into an approach to child abuse that seeks to avoid past over-reactions, but it is quite likely that in the future they will miss some of its new manifestations, and again be blamed for a lack of vigilance. Society remains deeply troubled and ambivalent about child abuse.[10]

The failure of most child protection investigations to lead to convictions or to stop abuse continuing inevitably led to their reappraisal, especially as being on the receiving end of an investigation is frightening and overwhelming to families, who can subsequently feel unable to trust their local social services and less confident about asking for the very help they need. Parents often feel a child protection investigation means their child will be taken away from them, although this is highly unlikely. Somewhere along the line, social services alienated themselves from parents who were simply not coping and needed support, including ethnic minority parents, who sometimes felt that a child protection investigation, because of police involvement, might bring an associated risk of deportation, as well as leading to great shame within their own community, particularly for mothers.

At other times, social services were far too easily manipulated by a small group of serious abusers who should have been more consistently investigated and assessed over a period of time, and where staff often over-compensated in cases involving ethnic minority parents for fear of being accused of racism. The difficulty for staff is that it is only possible to tell which parents pose the greatest threats with hindsight.

## Profile of Rikki and Ruth Neave

Six-year-old Rikki Neave died in November 1994 while in the care of his mother, Ruth. She was acquitted of his murder at a subsequent trial but as a result of his death and the life he had lived while alive, Cambridgeshire Social Services developed a new risk policy. Rikki's mother, Ruth Neave, had been in care to Cambridgeshire as a teenager, and had given birth to Rikki while living in a children's home – in fact while she was still bed-wetting as a 16 year old. Her own parents had committed suicide in a pact, having rejected Ruth all her life, and placing her in long-term care from the age of 2. Although she gave innumerable warning signs of the risks and threat she posed to Rikki, his plight was never properly understood. Staff energy went into supporting his mother and resisting her aggression towards them. The almost symbiotic obsession staff in Cambridgeshire social services had with Ruth Neave affected decision-making, although staff alleged that lack of support and guidance for them was just as important.

The case bore an astonishing resemblance to other high-profile cases in which children have died at the hands of a parent or a parent's partner. Yet as the Director of Social Services in Cambridgeshire said in his introductory statement to the independent report by the Bridge Child Care Consultancy: 'Staff are currently working . . . to secure the safety and support of over 340 children recorded on the Cambridgeshire child protection register.'[11] That is a lot of risk policies to get right at any one time, especially when the evidence in many cases is conflicting.

However much help they receive, some people will die in tragic circumstances. People with mental health problems kill themselves. Violent parents kill children. It is a mistake to start casting social workers in the role of criminals, guilty of greater crimes than the people who actually commit them. In Cambridgeshire, the 340 other children at risk apart from Rikki Neave needed an organisation strong enough to learn lessons and move forward, not one forced to retreat behind massed defences, warding off a hostile and permanently critical outside world.

Children are still being seriously abused and killed within their families. A fresh stream of young emotionally and psychologically immature parents, ill-equipped and under-prepared to cope with parenting a baby, will pose the same high levels of risk in the future, especially to very young and physically vulnerable children. The threat posed to children by some parents with mental health problems is also significant. A schizophrenic mother believed her child to be an angel who did not need earthly sustenance. She locked her in a cupboard under the stairs so she would not be sullied by contact with humans. The child, aged 6, received no food or drink for some days until she was found.[12] Many child protection tragedies repeat themselves, and sometimes it can seem as if the lessons are never learned.

These lessons include the following key points:

- staff should beware of being too optimistic (Tyra Henry inquiry);
- parents can lie and deceive, and social workers have to guard against being manipulated (Kimberley Carlile and Jasmine Beckford inquiries – Jasmine's social worker tried unsuccessfully to visit her 78 times before she died);
- professionals across agencies should share all information (all cases);
- staff should be prepared to doubt their own assessment and to reassess, if need be using an independent assessment (many cases);
- children themselves should be spoken to and listened to (the Fred and Rosemary West case);
- sometimes the people who know what is going on are not office-based professionals, but local workers on the ground like housing estate officers, relatives, neighbours and day care workers (many cases).

The number of children killed by a parent in the UK continues to fall. In 1974, 243 children were killed. By 1988, this had fallen to 112. The figure is now under 100, although what is not recorded is how many potential deaths have been saved by improved medical techniques at the point of admission to casualty or A&E Departments.[13] The UK child protection system is renowned internationally as one of the safest.

## Profile of Shaun Anthony Armstrong

On his thirty-second birthday, Shaun Anthony Armstrong sexually assaulted and killed a 3-year-old girl, Rosie Palmer, in Hartlepool. She had gone out to buy an ice cream from a van about 40 yards from her home only to be raped and murdered by Armstrong. The van had stopped outside his house, and he bought her the ice cream. Armstrong pleaded guilty to sexual assault and murder at Leeds Crown Court in 1995 and was sentenced to life imprisonment.

The seeds of what happened were sown early in Armstrong's life. His father was in fact his grandfather, and his mother was 18 when she gave birth to him as a result of this incestuous relationship. After an isolated early childhood, his mother started to sexually abuse him when he was 7, and this abuse progressed to full sexual intercourse when he was 13. He saw various psychologists and psychiatrists as a child. After leaving school, he joined the Navy but was discharged as unfit, and then had a series of temporary jobs. He was frequently convicted of burglaries, thefts and dishonesty offences. Aged 22, he tried to commit suicide, and then had a number of psychiatric assessments and admissions to psychiatric units in his twenties and early thirties. The attempted suicides continued. He also had a drink and drugs problem. It was alleged he sexually abused more than one young girl before he killed Rosie Palmer. His attempts to take his own life continued in Wakefield Prison after he had been sentenced to life imprisonment.

An independent panel of inquiry found that local mental health services had not cared adequately for Armstrong during the critical years preceding Rosie Palmer's murder, but that her death could neither have been predicted nor prevented.[14] Rosie's mother, Beverley Palmer, unsuccessfully sued the health authorities responsible for Armstrong's care. She claimed Armstrong warned on many occasions that if he was released from hospital, he would kill a child. It is possible that if the criminal intelligence about Armstrong's history of sexual offences and his statements in hospital to nursing staff had been shared between the hospital, the police and social services, there might have been a greater realisation of what he might do.

One in 3 child murders are committed by adults with mental health problems, most within the family. Whatever happened to Shaun Anthony Armstrong as a child destroyed not only his life but Rosie Palmer's and those who cared about her. Like many other child abusers, Armstrong was abused as a child and began abusing others at the same time as he was being abused himself. The two went hand in hand. He needed help as a child with unrecognised mental health problems and then as a young abuser. The only help Rosie Palmer needed was for Armstrong to be contained or cured before he met her. Her mother, Beverley Palmer, like Armstrong, attempted suicide on ten occasions after Rosie's death, through sheer grief.[15]

## FACTITIOUS OR FEIGNED ILLNESS: MUNCHAUSEN'S SYNDROME BY PROXY

While cases like Armstrong's reveal a strong inter-generational theme and a blatant deterministic set of factors, other child protection cases are more subtle. Too much attention can be paid to what seems obvious. As in many criminal investigations, the wrong adult can be accused, and the abuser of a particular child turns out to be someone nobody suspected. In other cases, such as when a young baby develops breasts in a way that can only have been caused by abusive over-stimulation, evidence is usually lacking and the management of cases has to be sophisticated. Some young babies develop breasts because of high hormonal levels, and hormonal imbalance has to be eliminated as a cause before the possibility of abuse can be investigated.

Factitious illnesses in a child abuse context involve the misuse of children by adults who want to gain attention for themselves. For example, a child can be slowly poisoned over a period of time, all because a parent wants attention for themselves and repeatedly takes the child to hospital to achieve that objective. Similarly, a parent might manipulate the dosage of a drug given to a child for medical reasons, forcing the child to take much higher doses which cause powerful adverse side effects. Undetected poisoning by dangerous mothers is not new. One of the nineteenth century's most prolific murderers, Mary Ann Cotton, poisoned three husbands and more than a dozen of her children in County Durham. She was executed in 1873.

## FACTITIOUS ABUSE AND RITUAL ABUSE CASES IN NOTTINGHAMSHIRE SOCIAL SERVICES

Nottinghamshire social services' handling of child protection work has a high-profile history. In the late 1980s, along with social workers in Rochdale and Orkney social services, some of their social workers thought they had uncovered evidence of satanic abuse, in which children were being systematically abused in cult rituals. The social workers clearly believed in what they were doing. Some were accused of being religious fanatics who saw the Devil everywhere. This was far-fetched, even though the Deputy Director at the time, Andy Croall, was a committed evangelist and had to resign over comments on abortion he made on a TV programme. But a joint inquiry report written in June 1990 by a joint team of social work and police staff for the Chief Constable of Nottinghamshire and the then Director of Nottinghamshire social services, David White, came to the conclusion that the 'Broxtowe case', as it was known, although a case of grotesque multi-generational sexual abuse of a number of children within an extended family, did not contain any evidence of satanic abuse or witchcraft.[16] Staff from the department and the police were commended by a judge and others for the quality of their work undertaken in the initial investigation and response. This resulted in words of praise in the House of Commons from the then Prime Minister, Margaret Thatcher.

The social workers involved were unduly influenced by a half-baked American therapist who had lectured them on what he saw as widespread international satanism. This man turned out to be an ex-FBI officer with no medical or educational background and no formal qualifications. It is likely he had picked up his ideas from the American conference circuit, on which in 1986 and 1987 a number of therapists were describing patients reporting recovered memories of satanic abuse. When subsequently contacted, the American authorities were surprised at how seriously this man had been taken in Nottingham. He went on to brief the foster parents about satanic indicators they should look out for, as they were looking after the children involved, who had originally been taken into care as a result of sexual abuse. The foster parents then helped the children to keep diaries, and the children's diaries became the evidence of satanic abuse. Staff were right to have sought advice from a number of sources that might explain some of the children's behaviour. It was the nature of the advice, with the benefit of hindsight, that was too readily accepted.

The diaries contained stories such as 'babies being cut out of the tummies of female members of the family', 'babies being thrown on the bonfire', 'the family having dead babies hung round their necks', 'babies being stabbed in a balloon and cooked in the oven', 'a Highman living in a big castle full of sharks and boats, eating children', and 'a child being cut with a knife and being made to drink the blood put in a cup'. The social workers took the view that the children must be believed whatever they said. This was hard to square with the fact some children at least would be dead as a result of the alleged cannibalism and multiple murders, but no child was ever reported missing in linked circumstances, and no corroborative evidence was ever found. The joint executive team report concluded that in taking the children's diaries at face value, social workers had ignored other influences upon the children, ignored the fact that the foster carers had been asking the children leading questions in helping them write their diaries, and showed little understanding of the 'suggestibility' of children as young as 3 years old who had already been grossly sexually abused. The children had been sadistically sexually abused, but they had not been abused satanically or ritualistically.

Ironically, the cases were evidence of a professional cult or fad, a cult about a cult in fact. As had happened in Cleveland and other places, faced with a sceptical and hostile public, social workers tended to overstate the extent of abuse in order that it might be taken more seriously. Diagnostic over-exuberance in Nottinghamshire was made to appear worse because other local authorities went around freely quoting what had happened there to help justify their own interventions. In 1994, in a study commissioned by the government, Dr Jean La Fontaine also found no evidence of satanic ritual abuse in the UK.[17] The arguments about the reality of recovered memories of sexual abuse, so called 'memory wars', go on, making it hard to be level-headed about child protection work.

The weakness of child protection arrangements in Nottinghamshire was emphasised a few years later in 1993 when Leanne White, a 3-year-old girl well known to the department, died while in the care of her mother, Tina White, and the man she lived with,

Colin Sleate. An internal review led by the then Deputy Director Stuart Brook, *Strong Enough to Care?*, published in July 1994, found a dire state of affairs in the social services department which required urgent remedial action, on top of serious errors of judgement in its handling of the White case.[18] The Director, David White, and the Chair of Social Services, both resigned. Problems identified included an insular culture, low standards, low expectations, a lack of training programmes, a reorganisation that was still not completed after several years, a high level of involvement by councillors in operational work which led to a confusion about who was really in charge, and a department that lacked a sense of leadership and strategic direction. On the plus side, after the Broxtowe case, White had set in train formal arrangements to ensure that any subsequent investigations into cases of ritual abuse were considered by senior managers in the police and social services jointly.

As a result of the *Strong Enough to Care?* report, an action plan was put in place, seeking belatedly to de-politicise and re-professionalise the department. Eighteen months later, Department of Health inspectors returned to find the department in the process of healing itself and growing up. The Children Act, bypassed before, was being implemented. Investigations and assessments were being handled properly, and case recording and supervision arrangements were in place. The department was working in partnership both with parents and with other agencies. In many ways, this had been a modern parable about life in social services over the previous decade. By 1996, whatever the excesses of the mid- to late 1980s and early 1990s, most social services departments had become realistic. Nottinghamshire social services, famous in the early 1980s for its pioneering community development work, was getting its pride back, and was again carrying out vanguard work in areas like family support.

Over a 13-year period, events in another case in the county illustrate the complexities of child protection cases and the difficulties staff face at the time, which can be distorted as well as illuminated by hindsight. In 1986, Celia Beckett poisoned and murdered one daughter, although the cause of death at the time was recorded as acute bronchitis. After this child's body was exhumed in 1994, traces of anti-depressant tablets were found in her body and Beckett was convicted of her manslaughter. She was also convicted of poisoning and cruelty to a second child. She was found not guilty of causing grievous bodily harm to a third child who died in 1991 as a direct result of severe disabilities acquired for no known reason in 1984 while in Celia Beckett's sole care.

At Beckett's trial, social services and the police were accused of a 'catalogue of errors'. Like other mothers who go through with threats that are often dismissed by social workers as fantasy, Celia Beckett had threatened to kill her children on a number of occasions. Similarly, she had asked for her children to be taken into care, but as in the case of Rikki Neave in Cambridgeshire, the advice went unheeded. It is easy to look back or look on in anger, but at the time, much less was known about Munchausen's syndrome than now. There was a different professional knowledge base in the 1980s. The medical evidence at the time was unclear. Above all, Celia Beckett seemed an inadequate parent, not a bad parent. The staff involved all the way through were conscientious and always acted in good faith. This case was a learning curve for the department, a process matched elsewhere. Blaming the participants can paralyse a much wider group of staff and agencies and even stop the social care profession as a whole from moving forward. Putting even the most distressing events down to experience and learning from them is much more likely to lead to service improvement. The county council acknowledged its mistakes openly, and talked positively about how it had already started to rebuild its child protection service. This up-front approach, compared with its defensive handling of past cases, helped to restore public confidence.

## CHILDREN IN NEED

The Children Act, introduced in 1991, established the key concept of 'a child in need'. Ever since, the definition of what 'need' means in this respect has been left either to professional or judicial interpretation. The tension about whether a child is in need or not is played out daily between professional staff in different agencies. Teachers will refer one child, whom social workers then say does not fit the criteria for help. Social workers will carry out a child protection investigation on another child, which teachers then criticise for over-reaction, and undermining the trust they are trying to build up with the family. Health visitors will over-inflate a family's needs because they think this is the only way to ensure resources are obtained. Agreement is hard to reach, but it is clear that many children in need are properly referred to social services who cannot help because of a shortage of resources. Psycho-social screening of children in nursery or primary school can begin to identify children in need, who then need to be subject to a period of sustained observation, the detail as well as the objectives being shared with parents.

Children with a range of complex emotional and behavioural problems currently represent the biggest challenge to social services, as well as to schools and parents. They are children who, while they may indeed need care, have a more immediate need for containment and control. These are the children who their carers cannot cope with, either at home or at school. Their behaviour can include fire-raising, destroying property, physically and verbally attacking carers, repeated thefts, constant running away, bullying and deliberate self-harm. Some 16 per cent of 7–8 year olds in the UK have attachment deficit disorders; 10–20 per cent of children experience emotional difficulties such as depression and anxiety.[19] Some 10–15 per cent of children behave aggressively. In 1995–6, 13,581 children were excluded from secondary schools.[20] However, as a nation we do not collect comprehensive statistics on the numbers of children in need. The Family Policy Studies Centre estimated there may have been as many as 400,000 children in need in the UK in 1996. It is a scandal that we do not know, and are not planning, how this number, if it is accurate, can be reduced. When education support programmes are put in place, exclusions from school can be reduced to a minimum. In one or two areas of the country, secondary head teachers have collaborated to offer places to all children on the threshold of exclusion, thus operating a 'no-exclusion' policy.

While there is nearly always an underlying set of reasons why a child behaves badly, few parents or professionals are able to change things for the better. As with terrorism, the underlying causes of a crisis are overshadowed by the shocking nature of immediate incidents. A number of children either leave home early and effectively disappear by agreement at 15 or 16, or come into care (as children looked after), when it is difficult for the local authority to find a satisfactory placement. Placements that are available are often both unsuitable and exorbitantly expensive, costing between £1,500 and £2,500 per week per child at 1996–7 prices – at least six times the cost of sending a child to Eton! Residential help is best given at a young age in a therapeutic community; 2–3 years' intensive help for a highly disturbed child at the 5–10 age, before defence mechanisms become too strong, or acting-out behaviour becomes too entrenched, may enable the child to resume normal development as a teenager, as long as the parents have changed too.

Where long-term therapy is provided for children whose problems have been correctly diagnosed, the prognosis is much improved, but being able to match the child, the resources and the right treatment is rare. Most workers in the field are concerned about the increased intensity of childhood disturbance they see, at an ever-younger age. It has not helped that a whole range of back-up services for young people, such as youth services, have been savagely cut during the last five years. The community education budget in Derbyshire for example was cut from £15 million in 1994 to £6 million in 1996. Youth services, like many back-up health and education services, are not mandatory services, so are often among the first services to go when money is tight. The increasing number of children excluded from school may be leading to higher levels of youth crime.[21] As a society, we are in the process of stacking up an increasing number of disturbed adults for the next century, if some of today's 14- or 15-year-old psychotic children are anything to go by.

The other main group of children in need is children with disabilities. As neo-natal care improves, children are being born who would not have survived in the past, but sometimes they are born with multiple disabilities. As a result, the child and family may need lifelong support. Long-term residential commitments become unavoidable if an infrastructure of community services is not in place. Parents and carers would usually like health education and social services to work more closely together in a properly co-ordinated service. It is amazing how some parents on their own cope with more than one child with a complex disability like Asperger's syndrome or autism, when it would take an entire staff group to carry out the same level of care in a residential setting. However, many of those same parents are at permanent breaking point.

### Julia's story

Julia's life has been hard. Her mother died when she was 10. Her first marriage broke down. She looks after her father, a dour miserable old man, who lives nearby. Julia's second marriage is strong, and it needs to be. Two of her three children have a chromosomal abnormality affecting the tenth and seventeenth chromosomes, which affects the development of the brain and leads to the collection of behaviours often described by the umbrella term 'autistic'.

Both Michael, 17, and Paula, 11, had major heart operations soon after their first birthdays. After Michael was born he had numerous tests but no recognised abnormality was detected and it was decided that he had suffered brain damage at birth, of no genetic significance. The worst moment of Julia's life was when, in an off-hand and callous way, doctors told her that Paula, her third child, also had the same characteristics which were later found to be an inherited chromosomal abnormality. No-one quite knew what to say. Nurses darted out of sight. For some time Julia could barely look at Paula. In between Michael and Paula, Joe was born. He is a healthy lad, now 13, who seems unaffected by the chaos around him at times. He loves his brother and sister with a fierce loyalty.

Michael has an obsession with water. Since his early years, he has headed for every unattended tap to turn it on and leave it on. The family house is regularly flooded. On a family holiday to a five-star hotel in Jersey, the hotel was flooded one evening when the extra carer Julia had taken on holiday thought Michael was asleep. Whereas at his residential school, Michael's bedroom door is alarmed, at home he is locked in his room at night. It is the safest thing to do. He does not need 24-hour supervision and care as much as second-by-second supervision and care.

Paula shouts endlessly and strips off regularly, regardless of who is around, which is difficult for Joe and his friends, and in time may leave Paula vulnerable. She regularly wakes Julia up at six o'clock in the morning by creeping into her bedroom silently, leaning over her then screaming 'Mummy' at the top of her voice. She can be heard across the street.

Julia's husband is supportive and plays his part, but 80 per cent of the stress falls on Julia. She has the added stress of dealing with professionals, who cause mini-crises by changing Paula's transport arrangements, just when she's got used to a particular driver and escort, or by making alarming statements such as suggesting future funding for residential care for Michael or respite care for Paula may run out. Julia's circle consists of wonderful friends and insensitive professionals.

All of Michael and Paula's birthdays are painful for Julia, because she can see the gap between how they are, and how they could have been, widening. But Julia rarely despairs. She is now a governor of Paula's school, and a campaigner for better local services. Her children have survived beyond their original life expectancy, and though there have been many traumas, Julia has survived too!

The general public have mixed feelings about children with disabilities, apart from supporting glitzy showbiz-led appeals like the BBC television Children in Need appeals which say as much about the British love of showbiz as anything else. One of the authors was recently sent a chain letter appealing for compliments slips to be sent on to a 7-year-old boy who allegedly had terminal cancer and wanted to achieve an ambition of being included in the *Guinness Book of Records*. On further checking, the local authority where he supposedly resided found that he did not exist, although such a boy had died of cancer at the same address several years before. Since the real boy's death, his family were plagued by malicious mail, business cards and now thousands of unwanted compliments slips. The British are basically a caring nation, but with a nasty underside.

## CHILDREN IN CARE

Children in care are now called children 'looked after'. The big question is just that, whether society's most vulnerable children are indeed being looked after properly. Social services have to act in the best interests of the child at all times, according to the paramountcy or 'the welfare of the child' principle. Some authorities fund a children's rights officer to independently oversee the quality of care they provide.

Compared with the general population, children in care are:

- 10 times more likely to be excluded from school;
- 10 times more likely to attend a special school;
- 4 times less likely to go on to further education;
- 12 times more likely to leave school without qualifications;
- 60 times more likely to join the ranks of the young homeless;
- 50 times more likely to be sent to prison;
- 88 times more likely to be drug abusers;
- 4 times more likely to suffer from mental health problems;
- their own children are 66 times more likely to need public care.[22]

The intention of children's legislation from 1948 onwards has been that each child in care should have their own social worker, to act as a good parent would throughout a childhood. In practice, children are in care today for much shorter periods, rarely for longer than five years, and usually starting in adolescence rather than as a young child. In 1996, 51,000 children were in care, down from 99,000 in 1981, and this figure now seems stable.[23] Thus, 1 in 250 children in the UK are therefore likely to be in the care system at any one time. It is still common for a child to have 3 or 4 social workers while in care, and sometimes no social worker at all. Some children in care never have their own social worker, for instance if their case is 'unallocated' or only dealt with on a duty basis. Children do best if their period in care does not exceed six weeks. Few children return home after longer away. Children who go back home after a period in care stay there longer than children who move on from short-term care to a longer-term care placement.

Over the last ten years, children's homes have been closing, either because of intolerably high costs, because children need more specialised placements than general children's homes or because the physical location of the home was in the middle of a residential area and life for the neighbours became intolerable. That of course is just where a children's home should be situated in practice, so that children in the care system grow up alongside other children, but the cumulative impact of high noise levels and dramatic incidents are often too much for local residents.

Children in children's homes do get blamed for everything that goes wrong in a community including car crime and burglary, which lets other thieves off the hook. Explosive mixes of children have made some establishments unmanageable, and abuse scandals have damaged public confidence in the care system which was low to begin with. In another twist, men are being deterred from entering residential work, and possibly from entering voluntary activity such as the Scout movement, through fear of being on the receiving end of an abuse allegation.

Though not as fashionable as foster care, and much more expensive, a residential placement remains the best placement for some children. For example, a child who has been sexually abused within their family may not wish to live in another family for the time being. Dwindling specialist residential provision denies choice to many children in need. As with other types of social services, residential care for children is crying out for greater co-ordination and funding at the national level. Without this, and without greater checks on owners and proprietors of small children's homes, unscrupulous operators can quickly set up private children's homes to make a quick buck from local authorities desperate for placements. In the worst examples of this, unqualified staff with poor skills and low values are paid a pittance.

The majority of children in care are now placed in foster care. This trend primarily reflects a continuing fall in the numbers of children in care, and slightly increased recruitment of foster carers. There are signs this trend is levelling out, in that the number of children in care nationally has plateaued and not enough people are coming forward to foster. Foster carers for hard-to-place children are the hardest of all to recruit. Most local authorities have specialist fostering schemes for children with challenging behaviour or high support needs, including paying salaried foster carers between £400 and £500 per week, paid on the basis it is a full-time job far exceeding the time and effort put into child care by parents in an average family. It is without doubt one of the hardest jobs in British society. It is no surprise that many foster care placements break down, when there's usually just one choice of placement for whichever child happens to need it at the time. A successful matching requires more choice and more preparation. On its own, foster care cannot deal with multiple problems. Expectations of foster carers are often far too high, with social workers seeing them as a 'magic solution'. A lack of educational provision for young people looked after who are often excluded from school as well places an additional strain on fostering placements when the child is around all day long and the carer never gets a break.

Trends in adoption are more in the spotlight since the shortage of babies available for adoption became so pronounced. Under 6,000 adoption orders were made in 1995, whereas in 1976 there were 17,000. Of those, just under 400 orders were for babies, compared with 3,600 in 1976.[24] Within the dramatic decline in the number of children needing adoption, the decline in the number of babies available is spectacular, in turn leading to desperate disappointment for childless couples wishing to adopt. It also irritates right-wing Conservatives and their mentors in think tanks. In August 1995, in response to concerns about low benefit levels for single mothers, John Redwood suggested 'If you can't afford to feed your kids – give them up for adoption'.[25]

Adoption law requires adopters to be able to meet the needs of children in care. Those needs are often complex social, emotional and medical needs. Put crudely, it's not enough to be nice, rich or well-connected, although this can be the way couples adopt from overseas through baby-trading organisations operating between the

Third and First Worlds. Babies or young children needing adoptive parents are not a civilised solution to childlessness for infertile couples. Adopters need to have built up considerable child care skills, usually from parenting or looking after children in some way over a period of years, not days.

The rigorous assessment process potential adopters are put through, including several probing interviews and a number of personal references, carried out by specialist social workers who submit reports to an adoption panel, can only judge applicants on past experiences, not on how they will cope in future. Assessing the present accurately is hard enough. After one TV programme on adoption assessments, relatives of one of the successful couples rang the local authority concerned to say the couple were not exactly the home-loving, tender and sensitive souls in the television portrayal, but habitual drunkards who knocked seven bells out of each other from time to time. Unsuccessful applicants, having exposed their most intimate family details to scrutiny by social workers, only to then be rejected, are often extremely bitter. Some go to the newspapers. Their protests led to revised guidance for adoption assessments in 1997, which enables prospective adopters to make representations against what they see as an unfair description of them, and to appeal against a decision not to approve them.

Once an adoption has taken place, the need to go on supporting the adopters is crucial. Placement difficulties can re-emerge after a lengthy trouble-free honeymoon period. It used to be thought that if you got through the first few months and broke the back of a child's 'resistance' you were home and dry. That is plainly wishful thinking: 20 per cent of adoptions break down, 40 per cent if the placement begins when the child is over 10. Some older children have gone back into care having been adopted after an earlier period in care. Post-adoption services were heavily criticised in a Social Services Inspectorate report covering a random sample of seven inspected local authorities.[26]

Post-adoption services also need to be made available to parents who adopt children from overseas. Although many social workers disapprove of overseas adoptions, the children are still children in need, and the numbers of such inter-country adoptions trebled between 1993 and 1996, with a dramatic increase in children being adopted from China.[27] In spite of these concerns, adoption is the most successful option for the small number of children in the UK who can never go back home. These children are usually not placed for adoption quickly enough.

## Mike's story

Mike was adopted at birth. Or at least at six weeks. He knew nothing of the details until he met his birth mother when he was 28, after the 1975 Children Act made it possible for the first time for adult adoptees to trace their birth parents. In 1976, those who sought to trace parents trod with caution and apprehension. Today, discovering long-lost children is almost fashionable. So is soul-searching. Mike's adoptive parents adopted him through the Methodist church in the late 1940s, before potential adopters were thoroughly assessed. His adoptive parents were in their early forties, but neither this nor their dreary suburban lifestyle mattered. What was unbearable from an early age was their marital conflict. They grew to hate each other. His mother communicated through him. His father didn't communicate at all, although he was sweetness and light, Mr Reasonable, to the neighbours. His mother spent most of her life moaning about his father. Like all children caught up in this not uncommon destructive domestic triangle, the sense of personal anguish and responsibility was heightened by his adoptive status. He must, he thought, be in the wrong place. He used to dream his mother was either a Russian princess, or the lady who came to the back door trying to sell Hoover bags and dusters. He found out he was adopted from a neighbour's child and felt a massive breach of trust, a clean break of the bond with the two people he thought he was literally a part of. From then on Mike trusted no-one. His adoptive parents' relationship problems heightened his teenage alienation. From the age of 11, he counted the days until he would be able to leave home at 16. Between 11 and 16, he was permanently angry, and now, looking back, aged 48, he remains angry. He still finds it difficult to get close to people or make relationships. Mike still craves attention, and his selfishness is always evident. Another side of him is the caring side, which started as a result of those years listening to his mother, and trying to advise her. On the surface he can be charming, like his father was, but his emotional scars are gigantic.

Mike's dissatisfaction with his adoptive parents was matched by a romantic yearning to be with his birth parents. The possibility they might have rejected him did not enter his head. His anger, that should have been directed with some sense of proportion, all went to his adoptive parents. Looking at it in retrospect, they did not know how to cope with his anger, which put even more strain on their own relationship. They had no decent advice themselves, either professional or of the common sense variety. After he left home, he saw them a few times before they died but nothing was resolved.

Mike did not tell them he met his birth mother and father, as he did not want to hurt them, and he was afraid the news would make them feel bad and they would in turn transmit that extra depression to him. His birth mother was pleased to meet him, even though his father, who still lived in the same village as her, was petrified his new family would find out and that his current life would somehow be threatened. Mike couldn't see how, whereas his birth mother immediately accepted him as part of her new family. She was married with two children who became Mike's half-brother and sister. You cannot start a childhood at 28, and after quite a lot of contact in the first year or two, they stopped seeing each other, although they exchange the occasional phone call, cards and presents. In those first months of contact, he and his birth mother had what was almost a doomed love affair. They longed for each other in different ways, and did not have the mother/son relationship boundary children grow up with. They did not know how to treat each other. For Mike the greatest relief came from finding out exactly why he was adopted. It helped to hear his mother was forced to relinquish him by her family and by her local community, who took a narrow view of pregnancy outside marriage in the 1940s. For her, the greatest relief came from knowing Mike did not blame her. She felt Mike had turned out all right, and had a better life with his adoptive parents than he would have done with her. Mike felt the opposite!

All personal stories conceal important social questions. Mike thinks his story shows that adoption should only be considered as a last resort placement, after an extended period of family support. He knows that many adopted children grow up happily, but he thinks the risks are too great for it to be advocated as a positive policy option without the utmost caution.

Children in the care system needing a placement have a right under the Children Act to expect social workers will take into account their race, culture and religious background in determining the best possible placement for them. Many children will be best placed with relatives within their own extended family, community and culture, and these same principles are usually applied quite properly to non-family placements. While all placements have to be assessed as safe from abuse and able to offer sustained nurturing in the long term before they can be used, race and culture are vital considerations in all placement decisions.

Just as residential care is the right placement for some children, placement with a gay or lesbian foster carer is right for others because of their own preferences or as a refuge. For example, a teenage girl abused by her father may feel safer in an all-women household. Being child-centred and being politically correct are often the same thing! Trans-racial and trans-cultural placements are also the right placements to make in the absence of ideally matched placements, or when for example a black child has been living in a non-black family for some years and the current carers represent security and stability, and those carers also positively support that child's black identity. Ideally, security, stability and identity-development can all be combined within the same placement, but a successful combination is rare. Perhaps growing up in the average contemporary British reconstituted family is no different!

## LEAVING CARE

Local authorities have various duties and powers to assist young people leaving care, until a child is 21 or finishes full-time education. Grants for after-care can be provided at any stage, which reflects what happens in many families. Research shows many young people leaving care face a greater risk of unemployment, homelessness and psychiatric difficulties than children leaving home conventionally. A 1997 Social Services Inspectorate study of six local authorities found that 75 per cent of young people left care with no qualifications, 50 per cent were without work, and 17 per cent of young women leaving care were pregnant. Nationally, 10 per cent of young people receiving severe hardship payments from the Benefits Agency are in care. 38 per cent of prisoners under 18 are in care, and 23 per cent of adult prisoners had been in care.[28]

Local authorities have tended to see their role as over once a care leaver has their own independent accommodation, but the need for after-care support is longer lasting than that. All young people leaving care need someone to keep in touch with, a base they can return to. Unfortunately, few are given that by the time they leave care, although many foster carers continue to provide unpaid after-care, thinking of the children they have fostered as their own children. One of the victims of Fred and Rosemary West, Alison Chambers, was in care in a Gloucestershire children's home. When she went missing from care, in 1979, aged 17, no special efforts were made to trace her. Fifteen years later, her body was dug up. She had been abducted by the Wests and callously murdered. The lessons of cases like Alison Chambers are that when children go missing from care, or when they set up home independently for the first time at 16, 17 or 18, social services must keep in touch with them and continue to offer support rather than cut it off. The longer a child is missing, concern should be heightened, not lessened. It cannot be right that services to care leavers between 16 and 21 remain at the discretion of local authorities, rather than being a properly resourced duty.

## PAEDOPHILES

Risks to children from paedophiles, which have always existed, have been better understood in recent years following the detection of some of the highest profile sex offenders. When the lorry driver Robert Black was arrested in 1991, a number of unsolved child murders in England were cleared up. In the USA, Johan Helsingius was thought to be responsible for between 75 per cent and 90 per cent of the child pornography posted on the Internet. While only a small number of paedophiles become serial killers, one man in ninety in the UK has been convicted of a serious sexual offence against a child by the time he reaches 40. According to Home Office figures published in 1997, 110,000 men in the UK have been convicted of sexual offences against children.[29]

The case of Fred and Rosemary West was one of the most macabre and appalling cases ever recorded in the United Kingdom. At least twelve young women were murdered over an undetected 20-year period, including some of the Wests' own children and girls literally taken off the street at random. The case illustrated that the divide professionals sometimes make between paedophiles who abuse their own children and paedophiles who abuse strangers is an artificial one, and a dangerous assumption to make during investigations. The West case only came to light because a police officer and social worker took seriously one of the West children's recurring statements that 'my sister Heather is buried under the patio'.

That children should be listened to is one of the key lessons to be learnt.

Rosemary West worked as a cleaner for Gloucestershire County Council at Shire Hall in Gloucester during the 1970s. It is possible Fred West worked as a gardener for the council. It is established that they targeted at least one and possibly more residential establishments for girls and young women in the Gloucester area during the 1970s, and possibly after that as well. At least one children's home, Jordansbrook House, was breached by the Wests, as Alison Chambers was living there at the time she went missing. Fred West managed to construct a monstrous graveyard in the basement and garden of a terraced house without being caught, due to a combination of tyranny, sleight of hand and exploitation of modern privacy boundaries.

It is important to heighten community awareness of the risks posed by paedophiles. The average paedophile has over 200 sexual contacts with children before being caught for the first time. Children cannot be supervised all the time, and they themselves have to take risks at times as part of the growing up process. Schemes such as Childwatch, in which local people are encouraged to report any concerns to the police, or Stranger Danger lessons, which are now taught in most schools in the UK, increase the capacity for self-protection against paedophiles.

It would be wrong to think a paedophile has an easily recognisable profile. Photographs of Howard Hughes, a paedophile in North Wales who in 1994 abducted and killed Sophie Hook, a 7-year-old girl while she was camping out in her uncle's back garden, made him look like a beast and a monster. In fact, even more disturbingly, paedophiles look like the average man in the street. Although Thomas Hamilton, the Dunblane mass murderer, operated through boys' clubs, and Frank Beck, the social work manager, through residential children's homes, we only know a fraction of what they did, and how they operated. While many paedophiles have a specific age and gender preference, no safe assumptions can be made. It now appears young people with learning difficulties might be at a higher than average risk, because of their inability to protect themselves.

Films that horrify the general public, such as the 1997 TV docudrama *No Child Like Mine*[30] which told the story of Kerry, who was abused by family members, friends of the family and a residential social worker, end up on paedophiles' shelves. What horrifies the average viewer will be viewed endlessly by paedophiles for personal excitement. The same applies to Mothercare catalogues, the statements of child witnesses circulated in prison, and fashion advertisements featuring young girls which are part of the trend towards the sexualisation and commercialisation of youth.

Social workers and police officers have to decide on a case-by-case basis who in the community should be notified about a particular paedophile. They will tell an unsuspecting woman with children if a known paedophile moves into a household without the partner being aware of the background. General community notification, so-called naming and shaming, in the way it is done in the USA and Australia, may satisfy the public but may also force paedophiles to go even further underground to evade detection and vigilante attacks. Selective notification of schools or clubs, and of immediate neighbours in special circumstances, is probably better, and is the practice in most parts of the UK under the general auspices of the Sex Offenders' Register. While sharing information about unconvicted paedophiles is more sensitive, because the accuracy of the information has not been tested out in a court, it is just as important because convicted sex offenders represent only a small proportion of the total number of offenders.

Paedophiles have infiltrated social services at all levels over the years. Some abusers have operated under cover as paedophiles for over thirty years before being caught, moving from one agency to another, sometimes moving frequently enough to deter a build-up of suspicions or questions in any one place. Many, such as Keith Laverack in Cambridgeshire and Mark Trotter in Hackney, were well-liked plausible characters adept at throwing suspicious colleagues off the scent. Information about their activities was downgraded and their own rights were unduly emphasised over the rights of children in their care.

Paedophiles in social work agencies sometimes also know the whereabouts of each other. Two directors of social services, when comparing notes, realised that a male social worker who was causing major concerns in one authority had obtained a job in the other authority in a team where two other male staff were under investigation following allegations of possible abuse. But for a chance conversation, the link would never have been spotted. Inside social work agencies, procedures need to be tightened up considerably. The Warner report, issued in 1992, on the issue of safer recruitment of residential child care staff, has been patchily implemented,[31] although Sir William Utting, reporting in 1997, found that basic recruitment checks had been tightened up by local authorities. The complacency about this is shocking. The 'rule of optimism' applies just as much to the way social services managers assess the risks to children from staff, as it does to social workers assessing the risks to children from their parents.

As residential homes close and more children are fostered, paedophiles will themselves adapt to a changed external environment and to new opportunities to infiltrate family placement networks. Roger Saint, convicted in May 1997 of a number of sex offences against children placed in his care, had fostered for at least five local authorities. Like Fred and Rosemary West, who were fined just £25 for assaulting a girl in the 1960s, Saint was convicted of indecency with a 12-year-old boy in 1972, but being caught and convicted did not interrupt his career as a paedophile.

Paedophiles themselves are usually victims of earlier abuse, as the Shaun Armstrong case illustrates. If children are to be protected, the paedophiles of the future need to be identified early and treated in far more vigorous programmes than are currently available.

## GUARDIANS *AD LITEM*

The 1975 Children Act first introduced guardians *ad litem*, following the Maria Colwell report.[32]  Maria Colwell was killed by her step-father, having been returned home by East Sussex Juvenile Court from foster care on the recommendation of a social worker. Maria's own needs were overlooked. Guardians were introduced so that children would have a voice in any court process about them. Panels of guardians were established in 1984. Guardians are appointed by courts to represent and safeguard the interests of children in public law cases. They are also required to advise the courts on allocating proceedings, in the time-tabling of cases and how best to minimise delay. There are currently fifty-four panels in England, including a number of consortia involving more than one local authority, and about 1,000 guardians, the majority of whom are independent fee-attracting social workers.

There are tensions between guardians and local authority social workers. Guardians fight for what they see as the needs of a child, although social workers responsible for cases do the same. Some of the battles come down to antagonisms about authority and status.

These tensions can often result in unduly extended court proceedings. The problem seems to be worsening the more the complete independence of the guardian service is advocated politically.

## FAMILY SUPPORT

Trends in social work tend to be cyclical. The virtues of family support are now being extolled, but in 1956 the Ingleby committee, set up to review juvenile court services, recommended a unified family service, including the establishment of family advice centres. Forty years later, the same policy is being lauded as if it is a new revelation. Much of what is now introduced with a fanfare as innovative draws upon the best of bygone eras.

There is a common acceptance amongst child care professionals that child protection services and family support services are two sides of the same coin, and that social services have to provide both simultaneously. Many families classified as 'child protection cases' are troubled by exactly the same issues as any other family, like poverty, loss, separation or divorce. Around the country a web of new family support services have grown up over the last five years, many of which challenge traditional ways of providing children's services. Services to women, who form the vast majority of 'parents in need', are being built up, although by no means everywhere.

In 1995, in the Earls Court area of West London, the Royal Borough of Kensington and Chelsea set up a family partnership team, funded by joint finance for three years. The area is multi-ethnic and in the first year of the team's work they supported families from thirty-seven nationalities. The team is multi-disci-plinary and is based in a local health centre. Social workers are called family workers as families find this less threatening, and the team has an education social worker and a health visitor. Work is short term up to a maximum of three months. Families needing help have much the same level of problems as families dealt with through the social services area offices. In a structured evaluation, 85 per cent of referrers thought there had been an improvement in family functioning or a lessening of the original problem after three months. Some 75 per cent of families themselves thought there had been an improvement and were no longer involved with any social services agency. Factors behind this success rate seem to be the team having a sense of purpose and confidence rare in social work teams, and the fact that education professionals saw the team as an education resource, health professionals saw them as a health resource and social workers saw them as a social services resource. Everyone thought the service belonged to them.

Over the last few years, Hampshire social services has used family group conferences as the main decision-making forum for individual children needing protection and children in the care system. Such 'search conferences' bring a wide range of extended family, friends, neighbours and advocates together, with professionals present only in an advisory role. These conferences are independently co-ordinated, which is expensive, working out at about £300 per conference. While police and legal advisers have a veto, Hampshire found that in 1996 the plan proposed by the family was refused in only 5 out of 150 cases. One child commented, 'For the first time in my life there was a meeting where I knew everybody.' One parent said, 'The family makes better decisions because they have the big picture. Social workers only have a small picture.' Long-term research from New Zealand, where the family group conference movement started, suggests that some plans adopted by families are not followed through, but in fairness the same can be said of many local authority-led plans!

In Powys, central Wales, family support services are provided by a network of home care workers (family aides) and childminders. In an area of 1,200 square miles, there was little point developing building-based services, especially as the only families who want to use these tend to be families living in the immediate area. The main service required by families is practical and emotional support. The service calls into question the need for expensive family centres and specialist staff. In one child protection case, where the immediate tension was a child who wouldn't sleep, twenty sessions from a family aide were given, understandably starting after nine o'clock at night. A sleep pattern was established which lasted. The service as a whole costs under £30,000 a year and supports twenty families at any one time, which means it costs about one-tenth of a conventional family centre. As a result of this and other intensive home care strategies, the skills of the home care workers and childminders have increased, which is good for staff morale as well as good in terms of producing a low-cost service based on early intervention.

Effective family support services are also provided by specialist voluntary organisations like Homestart, Newpin and Mellow Parenting. For the cost of a single child protection investigation

(£3,500 approximately at 1994–5 prices), a local authority can buy in seven Homestart or Newpin volunteers to intensively support one family each once a week for a year. Homestart and Newpin are organisations established by parents to support other parents. Volunteers are trained, and users of the service often feel more able to trust their volunteer than a social worker. They also see their volunteer more. One theme of their work is expressed by one parent who said 'only by talking to other mothers can you get the help you really need'. 'Positive' parenting classes can also help parents with a limited repertoire of child care skills. Some parents who used to hit their children but now are afraid to because they fear the police or social services will come round, have not learnt how to use authority non-violently. As a result, some 3 year olds, who have been brought up without any limits placed upon them apart from being shouted at, can play the same game with their parents, telling them to get dressed, when to hoover, and so on. Parenting classes can help parents set reasonable limits but to communicate much more with their children.

These services challenge the assumptions made by some child care professionals that they must be in control of social work for it to be successful. A changed role for professionals is itself a vital component part of any family support strategy. One of the difficulties establishing such services is that there is no clear taxonomy or classification of needs. However, detailed work carried out by Dartington Social Research Unit in a small number of local authorities found that where referrals and the needs they contain were studied in depth, services can be matched with needs. In one test site using this model, there were 40 per cent less children on the Child Protection register after one year. Twenty-two per cent of families were receiving more services.[33]

## YOUNG CARERS

The 20,000 to 50,000 young carers in the UK rarely want to be identified. Either the reason for caring makes them feel ashamed, or the reasons are kept secret from prying officials in case, as many young carers fear, they themselves are taken into care.

Young carers are not teenage babysitters. They are children sometimes as young as 8 or 9 who are carrying out the bulk of caring for one or more family members, either for a parent or for younger children. Sometimes the parent will have mental health problems, be suffering from ill-health or disability, or be caring only off and on because of drug misuse. The family will usually be scared to contact social services or anybody in authority, fearing the family will be broken up. Sometimes, the parents will be absent most of the time, and the young carer will be looking after the younger children in the family, getting them ready for school, feeding them, and putting them to bed. These are all tasks demanding emotional commitment as well as practical skills, and young carers often lose out on their own childhood and spend the rest of their lives forming relationships in which they compulsively adopt the caring role.

Social workers can offer support directly to families with young carers, or can arrange a contract for befriending through a voluntary child care or family support agency. Often, providing a sensitive home care worker is the best service, with the home care worker giving practical support to the young carer. Social workers will often be in touch with young carers without realising it. A referral defined as a child left alone, dealt with by warning the parent(s) not to do it again, may in fact be better defined as a young carer needing recognition and support. Often, through the need to manage workloads down to acceptable levels, and through the desire to appear unintrusive, there is a danger social workers gloss over many situations in which young carers remain unrecognised.

Just as social workers should not be judgemental about parents who depend upon their children, they should be equally careful not to romanticise what it is like to be a young carer. It can mean never knowing from day to day whether your parent(s) will be living at home or not, whether they'll be alive or not when you get home, or what mood your mentally ill parent will be in from one day to the next. That can be highly stressful for a child, especially if the uncertainty is corrosively long term. Some children cannot cope with such stress. If a care placement does become necessary, it is vital all children in such a family are placed together as they cannot afford to lose each other as well as one or both parents.

## YOUTH JUSTICE

Around 5 per cent of young offenders commit 65–70 per cent of known youth crime. For most young people, getting caught, arrested and humiliated in front of their parents and friends is usually enough of a deterrent to stop offending. Few go on to develop a criminal lifestyle, although young people may not grow out of crime as quickly as was once assumed. Zero tolerance of minor crime is all very well as a political posture, but given the criminal justice's system total crime clear up rate of under 5 per cent, lack of tolerance is rhetorical and to devote extra resources to it would be highly wasteful until detection methods fundamentally improve. The cost of running the current highly inefficient system was estimated by the auditors Coopers and Lybrand at nearly £17 billion in 1997. Less than half a per cent of total expenditure was spent on prevention, despite some successful crime reduction projects which reduced re-conviction rates for individuals from over 70 per cent for custodial measures to around 20 per cent.[34]

The public's main concern is with the hard core of persistent young offenders, but even this group is not a static population. Persistent young offenders change their pattern of behaviour very quickly, and some commit many offences in a short period of time, only to suddenly stop and adopt a new lifestyle. Because so little reported crime is solved, and a significant amount of crime is not even reported, an accurate description of the size and scale of the national youth crime problem is impossible. Crime patterns themselves shift constantly. During 1996 in North Yorkshire, there was a spate of thefts of floodlights from amateur football clubs. It transpired they possessed the perfect combination of light and heat for successfully and speedily growing cannabis! In London, drugs are increasingly dealt by mobile phone and home delivery, to avoid the risk of detection in public areas. Adult villains won't be too far away from the major young offenders, who themselves may use much younger children to front their operations. The fondness of political parties for hard-line policies such as military-style detention centres in the 1980s, which have failed repeatedly, illustrates the power of a dominant idea in social policy which can be pursued however illogical it might be, just like the so-called 'rule of optimism' in child protection work, when social workers convince themselves a family situation is considerably better than it really is. Youth justice services will be given an even higher profile with the creation of new Youth Offender Teams by the year 2000.

Use of youth custody for under 17 year olds in young offenders' institutions (formerly youth custody centres and before that detention centres) is falling, and is regarded as a blunt tool by both practitioners and researchers. A small number of deaths by suicide of young men in adult remand centres over the last few years has heightened concern about the dangers of locking up disturbed and disturbing young people. In hyping the dangers persistent young offenders pose to the general public, the risks posed by the same young people to themselves have been understated. Most social services departments have a policy of using secure accommodation on welfare grounds as an alternative to a remand to adult prison accommodation. This policy is in itself strictly policed because social services departments pay for the costs of a young person in secure accommodation, at about £150,000 per year per child, whereas the Home Office pays for prison remands and long-term placements of children and young people in secure accommodation after a court sentence under Section 53 of the 1969 Children and Young Persons Act.

There is a national shortage of secure accommodation places, although a government building programme will create an extra 176 places over the next few years. As with secure or medium-secure psychiatric units, siting a secure accommodation unit for children locally is an unattractive proposition for local politicians in the area. A local authority will look after other local authorities' most disturbed young people with a risk of something going wrong and a huge press outcry, and when it wants a place itself, its local unit is often full. The dubious ways in which young people who need secure accommodation are temporarily cared for in the absence of sufficient places, for example by using spare flats and security guards, is a national scandal in-waiting. Secure accommodation is only needed at all because of an insufficient number of specialist residential units for young people with high support needs. As a consequence, a tiny 10-year-old spree offender and a violent 17 year old from an urban gang can end up in the same small secure unit, living uneasily together.

Community youth justice work is delivered through bail support schemes and a range of community sentences which are classified as alternatives to custody. All projects have the underlying objective of diverting young people from the criminal justice system into a less anti-social way of life.

Examples of successful projects are caution plus schemes, the most successful being a county-wide scheme in Northamptonshire, in which young people are administered a caution in return for admitting guilt, and are then provided with an individually tailored community treatment programme; mentoring projects, whereby a young offender is befriended by a volunteer on a one-to-one basis (either a trained volunteer or a young adult who has matured out of offending behaviour); motor vehicle projects whereby a fascination with cars is legitimised through either repairing or racing them; or victim compensation and reparation schemes whereby offenders work on schemes to earn money to compensate their victims for an attack or a theft, and are confronted with the impact of their actions on their victims.

In 1996 in Hackney, East London, a Safer Cities project designed individual community treatment programmes for the twenty-five or so street robbers causing major local concerns. Informal feedback about such schemes has been positive, and while few schemes have been evaluated, there are signs that properly targeted intensive projects can achieve lower reconviction rates than traditional sentences such as attendance centre orders, which often deprive young people of liberty on alternate Saturdays without assisting them with the personal and social dilemmas they face, or making them more aware of their responsibilities to their victims and their communities. The Scottish children hearings system is based upon restorative justice, balancing the needs of victims and the needs of the offender with the requirement to punish. Other international models of youth justice, such as the Dutch system, also favour reha- bilitative or restorative projects. In France, an organisation with roots in the Catholic Church, Les Compagnons, takes on young people and trains them in a range of building trades, eventually offering work around France repairing churches. It was Les Compagnons who built the Statue of Liberty in New York. Organisations like the Young Builders Trust have started up similar schemes in the UK.

Youth justice workers are typically a mixture of social workers and probation officers either working in a joint team, or in a co- ordinated arrangement with a rationale for division of work, i.e. social services dealing with under-16s, probation services with 16 and 17 year olds. While a narrower 'justice-based' model was impor- tant in the UK in the 1980s for creating a shift in sentencing policy away from unnecessary and sometimes unfair custodial sentences, and to protect the rights of young offenders to a fair trial, youth justice services approaching the year 2000 need to be able to rigor- ously demonstrate the success of diversion schemes, in the face of constant political pressure for more sophisticated control measures like electronic tagging by satellite. The tags of the future may even be able to pinpoint the wearer to the scene of a new crime, although by then presumably the wearers of tags will have become more adept at losing their watchers.

High profile cases such as the Bulger case, in which the Home Secretary at the time, Michael Howard, unsuccessfully sought to define a minimum custodial sentence for the two 10-year-old boys, Robert Thompson and Jon Venables, who killed Jamie Bulger, play out before the public the policy confusion in the UK between care and control. At the trial, which was like a trial of dangerous demonised adults, both boys were sentenced to be detained at Her Majesty's Pleasure, which means until professional staff working with the boys recommend to the Home Secretary that it is safe and proper to release them. That section of the legislation emphasises the duty of care and rehabilitation to young offenders, even to child murderers. The Home Secretary sought to emphasise the control aspects of policy by defining a minimum 15-year length of detention, whether or not early rehabilitation was possible. The trial judge had decided 8 years was the minimum period of detention. The Lord Chief Justice had upped this to 10.

Mary Bell, the first child murderer of note, who was convicted and detained in 1968 at the age of 11 for the murder of two playmates in the school playground, was released 12 years later and is now happily married with a family of her own. 'Naming and shaming' children as killers who need to be detained for excessively long periods would be an unnecessarily expensive as well as a morally dubious youth justice policy. Children in care have often been demonised. In 1981, a 10-year-old boy in foster care in Dorset was called a poltergeist by his foster carers, because they thought he attracted the ghost of a dead drug addict into their house.[35] Poltergeists were to some extent popular contemporary figures. Supernaturalism was as topical in the late 1970s and early 1980s as satanism would become a decade later.

The bulk of work done by youth justice workers involves attending police stations as 'appropriate adults' under the 1984 Police and Criminal Evidence Act, to safeguard the rights of young people when they are cautioned or when they make statements; preparing court reports, usually pre-sentence reports; and implementing bail support programmes and community sentences.

Social services departments depend upon an effective youth justice team. If the police and magistrates have confidence in the team, their recommendations about cautioning and sentencing will usually be adopted. An inefficient team who network insufficiently will be on the receiving end of endless requests for secure accommodation placements, and will run the risk of their recommendations for more cost-effective community sentences being rejected.

In future, new youth justice agencies, and a new national youth board, will be established, whereby court processes are speeded-up with the police, Crown Prosecution Service and social workers working together. This might be the only way to eradicate the endemic adjournments in the current system in which lawyers are the only gainers. Like the young people they report on and supervise, youth justice workers spend a lot of time hanging around in courts. Such a new system could be funded by diverting funds from the Legal Aid budget. However, although few tears might be shed if lawyers suffered, children themselves could equally be the losers if their rights were sacrificed on the modern altar of 'value for money'.

# Chapter 5

# Does the community care?
## Social services today

Community care services to adults amount to three-quarters of all UK social services. Their sheer scale and scope make it hard to talk about them as a whole. The major community care service is to elderly people who become frail with age-related disabilities, but there are significant services to people with mental health problems, learning difficulties and physical disabilities as well as some smaller specialist services. While some services are highly expensive and professionally exciting, the most popular service is home care, in which home helps visit people to perform vital domestic work in the home and personal care tasks such as getting someone up, taking them to the toilet, feeding them, putting them to bed, and carrying out simple nursing tasks. The popularity of this service matches findings in the health service about the popularity of chiropody.

Community care is more than the sum total of what health and social services agencies do. Income support, housing, further education, and access to employment and leisure facilities are just as important. There is little merit in sorting out someone's alcohol or heroin addiction, if a job and somewhere decent to live cannot subsequently be found. Good primary care facilities, particularly GPs who will take vulnerable people onto their lists and support them intensively, are also vital. In some parts of the country, people with mental health problems continue to gravitate towards psychiatric units as their first point of call, just as drug misusers go straight to casualty departments or drug-dependency units if they go anywhere at all. In other places, GPs are providing a complete community care service on their own, with what they see as little input or support from other professional agencies. Other community health services which support independent living include community pharmacists. By making home visits to carry out medication checks and to promote medication awareness, they can prevent further breakdowns in health arising from taking too little medication or too much, which is a common problem for confused elderly people.

Community care services are being transformed in the 1990s. The status of social work with adults within the profession now equals that of child care work, which would have been unimaginable ten years ago, although some social services departments still regard child care social workers as the elite. The principles of social work with adult community care groups are exactly the same as child care work. Both services are based on comprehensive assessments and co-ordinated care plans. The same focus on no two children in care being the same applies to adults. In a residential care home, bathing one elderly person is not the same as bathing another.

Practitioners are becoming more aware of the overlap between services. The same person might have a mental health problem and a learning difficulty. Age and disability overlap. Drug-induced mental health breakdowns are common. Alcohol misuse is increasingly associated, or at least its connection is more recognised, with mental health breakdown, serious criminal offending, domestic violence and child abuse. A disproportionate number of parents with mental health problems cause child protection concerns. Because social services teams are virtually all specialist, staff may not see the wider connections in the cases they deal with. The same principle applies to services across agencies. Care managers, district nurses, housing officers and key voluntary sector personnel have to form close working relationships at the local level if services are to be as seamless as the public expect.

## SERVICES TO ELDERLY PEOPLE

Growing old is as complex as growing up. Today's elderly people look back on world wars and massive technological change in society. Some of those memories are desperately painful. It's not clear how middle-aged people today, some of them resisting the ageing process like mad, and still rock and rolling, will take to becoming 80 and 90 years old. The ageing process is psychological as well as physical.

Some 96 per cent of people over 65 live in the community, with some 73 per cent living alone (or with an elderly spouse). Over

600,000 day care places are provided, nearly 500,000 households receive home care, and over a quarter of a million people are supplied with lunchtime meals. 150,000 people over 65 are in residential care.[1]

Roughly half of people over 85 in the UK receive some form of care from social services departments. There are an increasing number of ethnic minority elderly people, especially in British cities, who rarely take up services, simply because they don't know about them. The more people over 65, the greater the need for social services in the longer term, because of the gradual loosening of family ties all over society, and because demographically there will be fewer young adults in the next half century to carry out the informal caring for elderly people which remains the main form of caring for people in the UK between 65 and 85 years old. The two biggest predictors of the need for care are age-related disability and the social isolation that comes from living alone. The greatest need for services comes in the year before death, whatever the age. Nationally, provision for elderly people is patchy. In some parts of the country, like London, pensioners and people with disabilities can benefit from a system of cheap and sometimes free fares on trains and buses, known as 'freedom passes'. However, there are no such 'freedom passes' in 10 per cent of the UK.

Nearly every old person who becomes frail or isolated would prefer to carry on living in their own home with support. Even without support, staying at home is almost always preferred. Sometimes, of course, elderly people refuse help, and it is in those situations that the local authority as well as the older person themselves are vulnerable. The law protecting adults at risk is far less rigorous than the law protecting children. The criteria for removing an elderly person from their home against their wishes, either because of self-neglect or a defined risk of abuse, are almost insurmountable. On the other hand, frail elderly people compulsorily moved from one place to another, for example after residential home closures, can find the move too much to cope with and may even die as a result. Old people are rarely adequately consulted about major decisions affecting their lives, whereas they would have demanded full rights of involvement to much smaller life changes just a few years before. When elderly people do die without anyone realising, as John Sheppard did in Brent, North London, the initial tendency to blame professionals for not knowing is tempered by a realisation that in certain circumstances it could happen to any one of us.

The body of John Sheppard, a single man aged 69 with no relatives, was found in his council flat on 8 December 1993. He had been dead for three and a half years . . . the tragedy was not that he died alone or even that he lay dead for so long before he was discovered but that he died unnoticed and unmourned. No one knew he had died, and no one pursued enquiries about him.[2]

Prior to the implementation of the NHS and Community Care Act in 1993, social work with elderly people was itself subject to institutional neglect. Work was often confined to dealing only with emergencies, or ordering a home help or a residential bed. A part of social services that was neglected for so long cannot be humanised overnight. Dismissive ageist attitudes towards old people can still be found amongst the professionals who visit them. In some American states, the rise in elderly people needing care has led to them being blamed for taking money away from services to needy children. It is possible that 'apocalyptic demographic' predictions of a rapidly ageing dependent older population in the UK have been overstated. Pinch suggests that 'some of these factors may have been distorted into a "crisis" by those on the right who are anxious to curb the welfare state'.[3] By doing so, insufficient weight and credence may be given to those social services which prevent high levels of dependency, like greater support for carers, and to medical developments which may improve the general health of elderly people in the next 25–50 years.

The financial regime for community care in the UK has a perverse incentive to use residential care, as it is cheaper than a 7 day a week care in the community package. This discourages the use of community-based options, although where these are provided, as in the Belfast intensive home care project, admissions to either residential or nursing home care can be significantly reduced. Residential care is better staffed as a result of tighter inspection regimes, and in general has become a safe if often mundane care option. The ratio of staff to residents in UK residential care homes increased by 38 per cent in the ten years to 1994.[4]

Despite these improvements, residential care should not be glamorised. It can reinforce dependency, limit rehabilitation from injury or illness, and undermine independent living. It can also be an unsafe environment, not just because MRSA (methicillin-resistant *Staphylococcus aureus*), *E. coli* and other 'superbugs' can be sources of widespread infection, but because elderly people can suffer subtle abuse from staff such as ridicule, refusal to grant wishes, and excessive sedation to maintain institutional peace and quiet, as well as verbal and physical abuse from other residents, especially residents with special needs such as dementia or depression. Behind improved exteriors, models of care inside can quickly turn from beneficial to punitive, particularly if the care regime is a 'warehousing' model where elderly people are processed through a series of tasks on each shift rather than the regime being a 'person-centred' model based on individual needs, coupled with a managerial policy of opening up the establishment to visitors, advocates and an empowered residents' committee. Elder abuse, like child abuse, is pervasive. Elderly people can be at risk of physical, emotional, sexual and financial abuse from relatives and strangers. Risk assessment in community settings is part of a good community care strategy. One of the prime functions of home care workers and district nurses is to keep an eye on vulnerable old people, to check as far as possible they are not being exploited by bogus tradesmen, burglars who return again and again, or the panoply of con men in every community. Appointeeship schemes are a way of protecting elderly people's finances. An independent organisation looks after an elderly person's money and pays all bills. Appointees should ideally be commissioned to carry out independent checks on the finances of all residents in public care, and all people with dementia living on their own and using community care services.

## Annie's story

Annie is 100 years old. She was born on the Isle of Wight and ended up in East London. Nowadays the reverse journey would be more likely. When she was in hospital as a young child with polio, Queen Victoria gave her a doll. Annie lives with her son and his wife. Her other son died in a motorcycle accident fifty years ago. Annie is a wheelchair user. Her son and his wife do everything for her, and have done since her husband Jimmy, who had been looking after her, developed Alzheimer's disease and died. Her son and his wife hope their own children will look after them, and they probably will because there is a family tradition of caring and good relationships across the generations.

Annie and her husband had refused all services offered to them, treasuring their independence. Annie was badly burnt on the top of her hand fifty years ago, and both then and now refused to have the burn treated, so it sits on top of her hand like a permanent festering boil. Her daughter-in-law, a lollipop lady, has to be careful not to knock it when she washes her. Annie's teeth finally rotted and fell out because she would not visit a dentist. She has to be transferred into and out of bed, and on and off the toilet, by a simple hoist provided by social services. Apart from the wheelchair, hoist and a helping hand Annie uses to pull the curtains, and occasional respite care in a local old people's home, no other help is needed. It is a long time since she has seen the family GP, and she takes no medication. She is partially sighted and hard of hearing, but refuses to wear glasses or her £300 hearing aid. Sometimes she loses interest in life and thinks it's time to die. Her son and daughter-in-law depend upon their social work assistant, Lorna. Her importance to the family is based upon recognising the needs they have as carers, and of being on the other end of a phone in a crisis.

Annie's care in the community costs very little. She has her needs met, and with minimal support, her family are happy to look after her. She resists easy stereotypes. She is stubborn, but gave up smoking at the age of 90 out of sensitivity to her relatives. She can get depressed, but likes watching horse-racing on TV and has a wry smile. She is mentally alert, even at the age of 100. In reading the files of older people, they can often be characterised in terms of their dependency and their physical needs. Annie is more complex than that. Her emotional needs are just as great, but she also gives out warmth and enjoyment to her carers. It is far from one-way traffic.

Pressures are increasing on local authorities all the time. Between 1988 and 1994, the numbers of National Health Service beds for elderly mentally frail people reduced from 26,500 to 18,200. The number of long-term care beds for elderly people reduced from 55,600 to 37,500 over the same period.[5] The scale of disinvestment in beds has not been matched by a growth in community services, so inevitably major cost-shunting has taken place from health authorities to local authorities. The incidence of dementia and depression increases with age, so the gradual but irreversible rise in the very old population brings with it a linked rise in demand for social care services. These long-term care services are known as continuing care services, and each local authority and health authority had to reach an agreement by April 1995 about what it will respectively pay for. The distinction is a crucial one, as health care is free, apart from prescription charges and visiting a dentist, whereas most local authority care attracts a charge or a fee. Placement in a health authority nursing home is free, but placement in a local authority residential home is means-tested and charged at full cost until the resident's savings have been reduced to £10,000, when the local authority takes over the cost. A charge may also be placed on the resident's former home, claiming all but the last £16,000 of capital. Older people feel aggrieved when a service they thought they had been paying taxes for produces the largest bills they have ever received in their life. Various inquiries have looked into this and more are planned, such as a new Royal Commission. The Rowntree Commission has proposed a new National Care Council to develop national standards for care, and to adjudicate on boundary disputes between free health care and means-tested social care.[6] It seems inevitable that future generations will have to pay for at least part of their care in old age, through insurance schemes or pension plus schemes as well as taxes. Between 1984 and 1994, 450,000 more old people became eligible to make some financial contribution towards their own care.

Who pays for continuing care does not have to end up as skirmishes between accountants. North Yorkshire Health Authority and York City Council have a flexible agreement for combined support to people who are near to death because of either illness or disability. During this period, the two authorities have agreed that dying people and their families should not be subject to a financial assessment or any dispute about charges. In other parts of the country, some health authorities define the maximum length of time for them they will pay for palliative or terminal care as 3 months, while others pay for up to 12 months. The costs which health authorities will not bear inevitably become local authority costs. Arguments rage about cost-shunting from health authorities to local authorities and vice versa, but it is clear that during the 1990s, there has been a massive reduction in the number of hospital beds at a far quicker rate than community health services have expanded. Once a patient is medically fit for discharge, she or he becomes a local authority responsibility. When the local authority does not make immediate arrangements for community services or a residential or nursing home placement, some health authorities have suggested they are simply providing a hotel bed and should charge the local authority accordingly. Local authorities will often argue the patient needs a longer period of assessment, or should

wait in hospital until the placement of choice can either be identified or funded. 'Delayed discharges' cause great friction, and battles
over responsibility are sometimes fought out in the pages of local
newspapers, with each side blaming the other.

There are other choices to be made. Britain aims high in its standards of care, with most providers of residential care committed to
providing single rooms for most residents, often with en suite facilities, and unit living environments, where units of no more than
eight residents live together separated off from other units in the
same home. This enables residents with special needs, such as
elderly people with learning difficulties, to be offered specialist care
but in a mainstream setting. Contrast this with some European
approaches, where large new homes are the norm, and shared
rooms are standard. History may judge this as realistic, and indeed
in Britain, large-scale providers of residential and nursing homes
are now looking to build 60–100-bed homes. Closure rates of
smaller homes have been dramatic in areas of high provision, such
as seaside resorts. Owners of small homes regularly warn or rather
threaten funders that they are being left with insufficient funds for
basic items like incontinence pads.

Meanwhile, one choice available to older people with healthy
bank balances is to move into a comfortable retirement complex or
'an assisted living facility' common in the United States and
Germany. Retirement communities, or continuing care communities, are a growth industry in the UK. The Joseph Rowntree
Foundation is building a new community consisting of 152 1- and
2-bedroom bungalows, a 41-bed residential and nursing home, a
restaurant, coffee bar, fitness centre, pharmacy, doctor's surgery,
jacuzzi and staff crèche. A 2-bedroom bungalow costs £85,000, and
the annual subscription or service charge of £7,700 a year covers up
to 21 hours of care a week at home, for cleaning, laundry, shopping,
preparing meals, gardening, dressing, bathing and giving medication. Rowntree is guaranteeing that the subscription or service
charge will never increase by more than 3 per cent above the rate of
inflation.

Decent warm housing for older people is an essential feature of a
local community care service, although housing authorities are only
under a duty to co-operate with social services departments, rather
than being under a specific duty to provide housing. None of the
181 clauses in the 1996 Housing Act mentions special needs. It is
likely the current Labour Government will introduce new legislation

to guarantee permanent housing provision for people with severe mental health problems, but there is little indication this duty will apply to other community care groups. In many areas, the only housing on offer is in unpopular and rundown districts which make people feel unsafe.[7]

In the longer term, lifetime homes, designed to meet the changing needs of occupiers, affording maximum accessibility, may become normal for mainstream housebuilding, supplemented at the high-dependency end by all-in housing and care services provided by specialist housing associations and private companies.

### Community-based preventative services for elderly people

There is a general trend in social services provision to channel and target resources to people with the highest levels of dependency and therefore the highest support needs. More home care is provided to fewer people. Services such as domestic cleaning and other practical support services are gradually disappearing from public provision unless they are part of a care package. These two sentences sum up the current problem. Over the next 5–10 years, more acute mental health beds will go, to be replaced by a mixture of day beds (known as partial hospitalisation), home treatments (whereby doctors and nurses stay with a patient at home for a few days around the clock on a shift basis), and crisis resthouses, which are like the old crash pads, somewhere to go for a while for people whose mental illness is not serious enough for a hospital admission. Most patients prefer shorter stays in hospital, and there is little evidence that people get any better the longer they stay in hospital. However, the public and the government will need a lot of reassurance that the new system will be safe.

The voluntary sector, traditionally a provider of preventative services through charities like Age Concern and the Red Cross, is not able to recruit volunteers in sufficient numbers to fill the gap. Volunteers should be in specialist volunteering schemes which give support and training, if the care they provide is to be of a high standard, and if they themselves are not to be placed in situations of some personal risk without realising it. The killing of Jonathan Newby, a volunteer with people with mental health problems, in a hostel in Oxford, illustrates the vulnerability of volunteering which the statutory agencies can rely upon to excess. Volunteers should never be left on their own.[8]

Preventative schemes for elderly people can be found in all parts of the country, but are rarely comprehensive in any one place. Most large local supermarkets will run a home shopping scheme for people confined to their own home. Tesco's, for example, have a catalogue with over 2,000 product lines, although it is only available in English. Homeshare schemes give carers a respite by using volunteer carers to look after a vulnerable older person during the day, or sometimes for short breaks. Care and repair, or 'staying put', schemes, assist older people to find reliable builders to carry out adaptations work, to arrange minor works grants and disabled facilities grants, and sometimes to carry out small repairs themselves. Carers' centres can provide support to carers which has an indirect benefit on the person cared for. As most community care is carried out by family members, the importance of carers' centres is yet to be fully appreciated. Many carers are older people themselves, so their need for support is heightened.

It is wrong to think of preventative schemes as meeting only a lower level of need in the community which in hard times can be dispensed with. Balance training can reduce the risks of falls in older people. As falls are one of the largest causes of hospital admission, treatment and subsequent rehabilitative care, balance training programmes are highly cost-effective. Routine installation of grab rails in new housing developments and estate refurbishment schemes can reduce the risk of falls, and can be included in construction specifications at negligible extra cost. A local database of adapted rented properties can ensure that all relet properties are matched to the needs of a disabled person, particularly a disabled older person who may be willing to exchange a flat or house which would be too costly to adapt in order to remain in the community. Home security projects, sometimes funded by local businesses, can fit strong door and window locks on elderly people's flats and houses and reduce the fear of crime, which is one cause of social isolation. Good neighbour schemes are hard to sustain with the pressures of modern life, but can provide better monitoring and early intervention as well as support, again, ensuring difficulties are dealt with before they become too serious.

Local residential homes, which have 24-hour staffing cover, can provide a hotline for local carers, particularly outside regular office hours when there is often no-one for a desperate carer to talk to. Residential homes are increasingly diversifying and offering some long-term residential beds, some short-term beds, some day care, and some respite care. By using their own resources as flexibly as possible, these homes can play their part in a community preventative programme. Flexibility will also be increased when expected legislation allows local authority homes to be dual registered as a residential care home and as a nursing home. An increasing number of residents in local authority homes are receiving high levels of nursing care, so new legislation would retrospectively regularise a situation that is becoming commonplace by default. Home-from-hospital schemes can arrange short-term support for people discharged from hospital, and voluntary organisations like the British Red Cross have shown they can provide these services at relatively low cost.

Resource centres for elderly people can act as a focal point for community activity, offering participation in a range of community-based events. It is possible for a small team of 2–3 resource centre workers to provide this service for a population of 100,000 people, by making extensive use of older active volunteers, and working together with local churches, pensioners' groups, over-50s' groups, lunch clubs, social clubs and tenants and resident associations. Events should stimulate interest including local festivals for pensioners, and outings – many schemes have been able to buy minibuses with lottery money. Befriending schemes and bereavement counselling work can be supported by small contracts given out by resource centre workers. Such a service, funded annually, would cost the equivalent of 4 residential beds. While such cost comparisons are only a rough guide, there is an added value of community involvement which can help reduce the marginalisation of elderly people.

New technology can also support preventative services. Some specialist providers are pointing the way. Community alarm providers are developing electronic monitoring systems which through the use of sensor equipment can monitor how safe people are in their own homes by sensing when routines have changed, or when the temperature of the home drops. By 2001, Tunstall Telecom will have developed the technology for a new mobile social alarm phone, which can be triggered anywhere, and whose position can be constantly monitored by satellite. The same technology that is being used to develop tele-medicine by the use of video contact between a person's home and a control centre, could also be used, with consent, to monitor particularly vulnerable people in their own homes, such as people with dementia prone to wander off, and people with multiple disabilities at high levels of risk. Small cameras can also be built into the alarms themselves. Caution needs to be exercised that the technology assists face-to-face work, rather than being seen as a way of replacing human contact.

On a larger scale, some local authorities are using satellite communication technology to improve access to transport for disabled people. Camden Council in north London is devising a strategy whereby all local transport like buses and cabs can be co-ordinated from a central point, and can be diverted to pick up people from their door and return them home.

## Meals-on-wheels (meals-in-the-home) services

Between 1 in 30 and 1 in 40 people over 65 receive a lunchtime meal courtesy of social services. Meals-on-wheels is one of the most traditional council services, usually cooked in central kitchens, often school kitchens, and delivered in vans equipped with hotlocks to preserve the temperature of the food. In some parts of the country, meals are delivered by voluntary groups, or integrated into the home care service.

Traditional council meals have been criticised for their lack of nutritional value and poor presentation – the meal often arrives at the service user's house too cold and with the elements of the main meal having worked their way into one another during the journey. The logistics of delivery rounds also means the meal arrives between mid-morning and 1.30 p.m. Recipients therefore have a limited choice of menu and time of eating. Community care legisla-tion emphasises the need for individual choice rather than individuals being given no alternative to a large monolithic council service. The traditional meals-on-wheels service is classically and negatively municipal.

Choice has been widened since frozen meals became available. The local authority will often provide a freezer and microwave and the meals supplier will deliver several weeks' worth of frozen meals, which either the user or a relative or a home care worker prepares on the day. As they are heated up in the home, they have the advan-tage of being eaten at the right temperature and at the time of choosing. This service is more accurately described as a meals-in-the-home service.

Supplying cooked meals in one form or another is an important social care service, helping older people live on their own when they are unable to cook a full meal for themselves. Recently, emphasis has shifted to the food hygiene aspects of the service, because of more stringent regulations set out in the 1990 Food Safety Act and EU regulations, and this in theory may limit the widespread use of informal arrangements. To limit community-based support in this way, when it has been in place for centuries and in many ways needs to be re-created, is bureaucracy gone mad.

## Dementia care

Dementia is the most common mental illness in older people. By the year 2000, roughly 1 in 13 people over 65 years old and 1 in 4 people over 80 years old will be suffering from a form of dementia such as Alzheimer's disease or Huntington's chorea. In younger people, multiple sclerosis and HIV infection can lead to dementia. The signs and symptoms of dementia can include changing moods or personality, memory loss, co-ordination problems, speech disturbance and delusions. Today, a new drug, Aricept, promises to delay the onset of dementia, although it is expensive and relatively unproven, and as such may not be funded by all health authorities. Within five to ten years, Aricept and a number of similar drugs may have begun to control the symptoms of dementia to such an extent that people currently looked after in residential or nursing home care might be cared for straightforwardly in the community.

Dementia care is a term coined to describe a person-centred approach to dementia, in which people with dementia are viewed as people instead of nonentities with half their brain missing. Dementia care requires changes in staff attitude. People with dementia are hard to communicate with. Working with people who have Alzheimer's disease, a progressive form of dementia, involves communicating with people who can on the face of it appear totally inaccessible. It is easy to give up faced with someone who screams without warning, who frequently leaves the place they're in, sometimes thinking they're returning to the house they were born in, and who has little control over normal bodily functions. Dementia is a form of bereavement before death. It would be all too easy to treat people with advanced dementia as akin to babies, who need total care, and where the carer is there simply to police and protect them. For carers, it can be hard to maintain high standards of care when looking after someone who cannot respond and who does not recognise you a lot of the time, but if those standards slip, it can be the first stage of a dehumanisation process.

In residential settings, the type of care being given to people with dementia can be monitored by dementia care mapping exercises,[9] which can then be used in training programmes with staff to ensure residents' lifestyles and routines are respected, and that their inability to express themselves at times is understood but not used as a reason to pretend they're not there. In one home, a resident with dementia would leave the home and try to cross a busy main road. One morning a staff member followed her, and saw her try to get into a parked car on the main road. From then on, an old car was parked within the grounds of the home on the resident's route, and each day she went to it and sat in it happily.[10] People with dementia are prone to wander and ideally need to live in a building designed with figure of 8 corridors and other navigation aids, so they cannot wander out into the street unnoticed, and so they always end up at the place they started out from, as well as being able to find their way around.

In community settings, new support services being developed include the use of Alzheimer's guide dogs, who alert the carer when the sufferer wanders off, and telephone reassurance schemes, such as the 'Mrs Smith's Handbag scheme' funded by BT in conjunction with Community Service Volunteers, whereby volunteers ring isolated people daily to keep in touch, and more general community care services such as day and night sitting.

Caring for someone with dementia is never easy. In the words of a carer speaking at a conference organised by Jewish Care, relatives have to learn quickly:

> I became a skilled psychiatric nurse overnight, a mother to my mother; a minder. A gate was placed at the top of the stairs, from the time we found her with the sleeves of a cardigan on her feet. The cooker mains were switched off between use, from the day my Mum had filled a saucepan to heat the water to pour over her hurting feet.

Carers within the family cope on their own, and as a result often make themselves ill. People with dementia can be violent towards their carers, either through frustration, delusion or as a direct result of changes in the brain. Carers develop their own way of calming the sufferer down, which might include physical violence back, such as biting, or even giving a favourite chocolate biscuit. The Carers National Association estimates that out of 7 million carers in the UK, over 4 million become ill themselves as a result of caring.

Caring for the carer is as important as caring for the person with dementia.

## PEOPLE WITH MENTAL HEALTH PROBLEMS

If parents who abuse their children are the most publicly loathed group of social services users, people with mental health problems are the most feared. An absconding patient who had threatened someone with a knife was described in local papers as 'knife nut at large', 'danger man on the run', and 'man who cut wife's head off', despite none of those descriptions matching the known facts.[11] For someone who is mentally ill, it's still more likely they'll be attacked than do the attacking. A diverse group of vulnerable people, some of whom are briefly ill after childbirth, or after a bereavement, or who struggle through life to fight against depression or chronic anxiety, have become muddled up in the public mind with a relatively small but growing number of patients suffering from treatment-resistant schizophrenia and other severe mental illnesses. One in four people will consult their GP about a mental health problem at some point in their lives. The prevalence rates for severe mental illness are not increasing. More worrying are the near-epidemic levels of depression and anxiety in the general population, attributable to a pot-pourri of social factors such as an obsessive work ethic, exam pressures, depression following redundancy or premature retirement, relationship breakdown or family dynamics.

Despite the general deterioration in the nation's mental health levels, there are grounds for optimism that new drug treatments may help people suffering from the most severe mental illnesses. When Christopher Clunis, a psychiatric patient for many years, killed the musician Jonathan Zito at Finsbury Park tube station in December 1992, concerns about public safety escalated. Other cases quickly followed, where patients with schizophrenia were discharged from hospital without an adequate care plan and supervision. Nurses and social workers lost track of them, or they refused to take prescribed medication. A number of serious incidents have taken place, and are still taking place, including random assaults and murders, in which a profound breakdown of communication between professionals has often been highlighted. The Boyd committee talked of 39 homicides and 240 suicides committed by people with serious mental health problems annually in the years up to 1995.[12] Several high profile inquiries, like the report into the care and treatment of Martin Mursell, have produced mirror-image findings.[13]

Martin Mursell, a 27-year-old young man who had been schizophrenic since the age of 21, killed his step-father and tried to kill his mother in a multiple stabbing in Islington, north London. He had been admitted to psychiatric units on several occasions, but lacked effective health and social services support in the three months preceding his violent assault on his mother and step-father. His care plan on discharge prior to the assaults was described by the inquiry as 'woefully inadequate'. However good his care had been in the past, that care had to be continuous to be effective. Six weeks after the Mursell inquiry was published, another patient discharged by the same health trust in Camden and Islington, Tolga Kurter, killed a neighbour in the street in a multiple stabbing. Despite the invariably bleak scenarios portrayed in inquiries, a new generation of drugs like clozapine and seroquel may significantly reduce levels of risk and violence within ten years. Of the first fifty patients at Rampton special hospital put on clozapine, 21 were soon discharged safely or transferred to lower security units.[14] Clozapine is expensive and has powerful side-effects, and it is not licensed for prescription outside hospital, but within ten years, it is possible that similar drugs will have been able to control the excesses associated with schizophrenia, and to be able to break the illness down into its constituent parts. Clunis himself, now in Rampton special hospital, sued his local health authority for failing to care for him adequately before he killed Jonathan Zito, but the Court of Appeal, in December 1997, refused his claim for damages. A community treatment order, had the legal power existed, giving mental health workers the legal backing to force him to take the medication which kept him relatively well and stable, could possibly have saved both Jonathan Zito and Clunis himself. A combination of tighter legislation, more effective drugs, and more resources for community mental health services, would support and contain the most dangerous features of severe mental illness. It is ironic that while psychiatrists supported the introduction of community treatment orders, psychiatric nurses opposed them on the grounds their professional relationship would be compromised by having compulsory powers, conveying the unfortunate impression of a disunited profession.

## Profile of Christopher Clunis

The Clunis inquiry report was published in 1994.[15] Like most inquiries, it pieced together information that should have been circulating between the agencies who saw Christopher Clunis over a period of six years. Similar retrospective collation is a feature of child care inquiries and does little to reassure the public that statutory agencies have organised information properly at the time they need to take action. In the late 1980s and early 1990s, Clunis had drifted through homeless hostels and psychiatric units in London, unable to care for himself because of paranoid schizophrenia. Clunis gave several warning signs of violent and aggressive tendencies including the use of knives in some potentially fatal incidents before he killed Jonathan Zito in exactly the same way.

In the years before the killing, several psychiatrists and social workers helped Clunis, just as others didn't, but his underlying condition remained a serious and disabling one. His case illustrates the profound difficulties mental health workers face in caring for people with schizophrenia. At times, he wasn't there when people called to monitor him. He often said he was fine when he wasn't. At times he was given the maximum allowable dosage of powerful tranquillising drugs sometimes known as chemical coshes, but this had little if any effect on his violent tendencies. The responsibilities community mental health staff had at the time, or have now since the Mental Health (Patients in the Community) Act 1995, implied the impossible, that staff could always track people like Clunis and intervene before the public were in any danger. However, in Clunis's case, it was clear by 1991 at the very latest, some eighteen months before he killed Jonathan Zito, that he required long-term support and treatment whether he wanted it or not. The question is why he was not kept in a secure setting.

There is more than one answer. One is that there are insufficient beds of the right type. This resource crisis means patients can be left in unsatisfactory conditions, especially if they are not demanding hospital admission. Another reason is that health authorities and local authorities tend only to make expensive residential and nursing care placements when a problem has become unavoidable, rather than when it is necessary. This is inevitable when budgets for care are cash-limited and needs have to be prioritised. The third and less defensible answer in Clunis's specific case was the bewildering number of psychiatrists and social workers temporarily responsible for his care over a 6-year period. While some were concerned, no one person got to grips with his psychiatric deterioration over a period of time and with the virtual inevitability he would kill or seriously wound someone. That failure to co-ordinate and organise care, to 'catch and carry' his needs across artificial boundaries like local authority and health authority catchment areas, quickly confirmed public fears that maniacs are on the loose now that the large psychiatric hospitals have closed and no-one knows where they are. Just as new trial drugs may at last lead to long-term reductions in violent and aggressive behaviour caused by mental illness, so new ways of organising community care services may prevent people from falling through the net in the way Christopher Clunis did. Time and again in relation to social services and its partner agencies like health authorities and education authorities, co-ordinating services properly would constitute a genuine improvement at no extra cost. The same can be said about many other services.

Chronologies like Clunis's make the 1960s' anti-psychiatry thesis that schizophrenia is related to family problems seem naïvely indulgent. The suggestion that in some way mainstream psychiatry involved human rights violations also seems far-fetched. Yet in the context of psychiatry up until the 1960s, the movement was understandable. The old 'bins' have virtually all gone now, but to go into them and see ward after ward of blank faces, drained of energy and adventure, cut off from the noise and chaos of normal life, was and remains a harrowing experience. A visitor could get lost in the grounds of a large psychiatric hospital, with their general stores, farms, post boxes (not that they were used much), and cricket pitches. The hospitals were societies within society. We will never know what abuses took place there. Some ex-patients defining themselves as psychiatric survivors would also say the treatment regimes were unnecessarily and unhelpfully draconian, and that alternative complementary therapies such as acupuncture, homoeopathy and hypnotherapy are still under-used.

The Mental Health Act Commission regulates hospital conditions, particularly ward environments, monitoring standards of safety, privacy, dignity and professional care. They report in general terms every two years to Parliament, and visit each local psychiatric facility at least annually, producing public reports which often require health authorities and local authorities to take remedial action. This has led to improved conditions such as women-only wards, important because of the degree of sexual harassment that

frequently takes place on mixed wards. The commission also monitors whether patients' complaints and representations have been
taken up.

### Profile of Tim

Tim is 29 years old. He has been an in-patient in an acute psychiatric unit for a year. It is his seventh admission since the age of 17.
His diagnosis is schizophrenia but this seems an imprecise label for
his complex emotional and psychological state, which is by and
large resistant to drug treatment. He is afraid to leave the closed
ward, apart from occasional forays around the hospital. It is as if he
finds the world outside as dangerous as it finds him.

Tim will probably never survive on his own. He will need in-
patient care or 24-hour support for the rest of his life. In theory, his
symptoms may quieten down when he gets older, but if this happens
it is likely it will be as a result of his being institutionalised somewhere rather than because he has recovered. He has lived with
mental illness since he was born. His mother is a regular in-patient
in the same hospital, although now she is living in supported
housing nearby. No-one will ever know quite what happened during
Tim's childhood. He seemed to have adapted to his strange way of
life until the age of 12. Before then, his mother looked after him as
best as she could, and when she was in hospital, Tim went to foster
parents. He was always alone, at home and at school. Like his
mother, he hardly ever went out. He never had a friend, and he
began to withdraw completely as a teenager.

As part of the inner world he has invented to get away from the
pain of the real one, Tim denies his mother's existence, even though
sometimes they occupy neighbouring wards. He denies he ever lived
with foster parents. He has invented a twin brother, who is always
about to visit him. His only relationships are with the ward staff
and a visiting psychologist.

Staff, including his social worker from the local community
mental health team, spend months gearing him up for another
discharge in another flat or another half-way house. Even though
the care plan inevitably fails when he quickly relapses, they have to
make the effort. In the old days, he would have rotted away in an
asylum, and never seen the light of day, but in reality, the outcome
today is little better.

A number of questions go unanswered. Is his illness hereditary?

Has he taken on aspects of the personality of his mother as a result of their own bizarre relationship as mother and child? Is a breakthrough possible, if staff only knew how? We know that some people with mental health problems do manage to break out of the straitjacket it imposes. But Tim never seems well enough to give his helpers something to build on.

## Community mental health teams

Community mental health teams offer assessment and treatment services to people with severe mental health problems. The most common way of organising CMHTs is by sectorisation, in which a multi-disciplinary team takes on the responsibility for a geographical area, including an admissions ward in a local psychiatric unit or hospital. Thus the management of hospital beds and community services is brought under common management by the same person, the objective being to stop patients falling through the net. Sectorisation also includes all GP practices within the sector.

GPs tend to work well with CMHTs, because for the first time they have access to a service which readily accepts their referrals. However, conflicts can arise because budget-holding GPs often want their own community psychiatric nurse, and tend to want to buy counselling services for patients on their list as a preventative resource. Tension exists between GPs and CMHT members, the latter often working with the most chaotic patients who are not on any GP list, who need intensive services rather than counselling. CMHT members resent the element of the overall mental health budget which is diverted in this way to less acute needs.

An evaluation of one of the earliest care programme approaches, in West Lambeth, London, makes sober reading.[16] Three-year programme results up to 1996 in respect of patients with marked turbulence and a history of violence showed no significant improvement in social skills or clinical functioning. These patients were on the highest tier of the Care Programme Approach, including being on the mental health supervision register. Sixty per cent of patients in the original cohort had been charged with violent offences and half the patients in the study had been victims of crimes. There had been a massive increase in demand for services, particularly in the use of hospital beds. A study by the King's Fund in 1997 showed that the psychiatric system in London is unable to cope with the demand for acutely ill patients, partly because the NHS funding formula does not reflect fully the links between mental health, poverty, homelessness, ethnicity and drug misuse.[17] In 1997, many patients are still living in grossly inadequate rented flats, with inadequate levels of community supervision and sometimes no care plan at all.

## Preventative services

The vast majority of mental health resources are still spent on acute care in hospital. The percentage of overall community care funding allocated to mental health has gone down in recent years. These two sentences sum up the current problem.

While a small percentage of people with mental health problems require the co-ordinated support and monitoring of a multi-disciplinary team, most people can be supported in the same way as any other group of community care service users. Supported housing, supported employment, drop-in services including café projects where people with mental health problems can go for social support and advice and information, are all important local resources, especially in cities. In more rural areas, the role of the professional nurse or social worker becomes even more important, because of the risk of isolation. Contact with people needs to be maintained, if necessary by assertive outreach work, which positively seeks out and keeps contact with people, so that signs of a relapse can be acted upon quickly.

Adult placement schemes are literally foster care for adults, particularly adults with mental health problems, a learning difficulty or dementia. There are over 300 schemes in the UK, some of which have lowered their starting age to 16 so as to be able to cover the transition between the services a child receives and the services she or he may need to receive as an adult. Carers are more likely to have finished raising their own children. A high number have worked in a caring profession themselves like nursing. Some 75 per cent are over 40 years old and 50 per cent over 50 years old. In large-scale hospital reprovision programmes, accommodation for long-stay residents has been made available in the local community by widows and widowers with rooms to spare. Adult fostering can greatly increase the personal care and self-help skills of people placed, and while not as cost-effective as foster care for children, is still a cheaper option than either residential care or intensive care provided in the home, although changes in housing benefit regulations have increased the cost to local authorities. In this respect, the recent Conservative

Government seemed to view a number of supported housing arrangements with suspicion, especially where three or more adults are looked after. Whether supported housing is defined as adult fostering or a hostel affects housing benefit calculations. The less housing benefit that is paid, the more social services departments have to top up the cost of the care element in the support. This is another example of one branch of government trying to out-manoeuvre another in relation to community care payments.

**Approved social work**

Under Section 114 of the 1983 Mental Health Act, local authorities have a duty to approve social workers 'having competence in dealing with mentally disordered people' and under Section 13(1), the approved social worker (ASW) has a duty to assess people 'within the area' for their admission to hospital, if appropriate. Section 28(3) of the 1977 National Health Service Act places a duty on local authorities to provide a social work service to hospitals in their area.

Approved social workers are co-signatories to 'section papers', along with either GPs or psychiatrists, which have to be signed before a patient can be admitted into psychiatric care without consent. The work can be high-profile as compulsory detention can be appealed to a mental health review tribunal. The ASW is personally responsible for each such decision made.

When social work teams were generic, many social workers were 'warranted' as ASWs, but as the standards for reassessment grew stiffer, only specialist mental health social workers could retain their approval, and guarantee to carry out a sufficient number of assessments each year to keep their skills honed. To be an approved social worker, qualified social workers must take a further 60-day post-qualifying course, including a dissertation and law exam, and meet a list of thirty-eight different levels of competency – the thirty-eight competency standard.

The role of the ASW may be one of the most neglected in modern social services. Many mental health strategies completely fail to mention approved social work. Local authorities have tended to provide low-key day care and residential care, avoiding the heavy-end mental health work carried out through acute and community mental health trusts. Approved social workers have lacked effective reference points within their local authorities, hence the recent trend towards developing community mental health teams including psychiatrists and community psychiatric nurses. This has helped ASWs to strengthen their practice and knowledge base, even if at times they have to stand alone professionally within medical teams that are multi-disciplinary in name only.

### Profile of Gilbert Kopernick-Steckel[18]

On Sunday 14 January 1996, in Croydon, Gilbert Kopernick-Steckel knifed his mother to death and then killed himself in the same way. Gilbert was a 36-year-old architect who had been assessed in 1980 at the Maudsley psychiatric hospital after a shoplifting conviction. A psychiatrist diagnosed him as having a personality disorder including a difficulty making relationships, but that he was unable to accept help because he saw psychiatrists and psychotherapists as negative authority figures. In the next sixteen years, during which time he worked mostly in Paris and Berlin, he had no known formal mental health assessment, yet in the days leading up to the murder and suicide, it was clear he was developing an acute mental illness requiring urgent hospital admission. He was diagnosed as in need of admission by his GP and a duty psychiatrist two days before the critical events, on Friday 12 January. However, they did not contact the approved social worker on duty. Instead they left various messages with receptionists. The potential urgency of the situation, which had been properly identified by the doctors, was not conveyed to the ASW who also needed to make an assessment before signing her part of the Section papers. Either a Section 4 (3-day emergency), or a Section 2 (28 days for assessment) admission would have been required, preferably a 28-day admission, given the extent of Gilbert's sudden deterioration and his open statements about wanting to kill his mother. In fact, the duty psychiatrist and the GP had both signed their parts of a set of Section 2 papers, indicating the danger Gilbert posed to his mother in particular.

Unable to complete the assessment because of a problem getting hold of the half-complete Section papers, the ASW passed the referral to the emergency duty team (EDT) covering Croydon for the weekend. On the Friday evening, they found out that Gilbert had voluntarily admitted himself to hospital. The EDT therefore did not pursue the formal admission. The sensible plan was to detain him on the ward if he tried to leave. However, the shift coming on duty in the acute psychiatric ward the next morning (Saturday) were not properly briefed and allowed Gilbert to go home when he asked to. The ASW was neither informed of the change in plan, nor of his return home. For the remainder of Saturday and the first part of Sunday, back at home, Gilbert behaved strangely but because the family had not been advised how dangerous he was by then, they coped as best they could without seeking to raise any further alarm bells. By this time Gilbert had been developing a progressively more acute psychotic episode for at least two days. Even Gilbert himself realised he needed to be detained in hospital for his own good.

On the Sunday morning, Gilbert asked the police to drive him to hospital and eventually he readmitted himself. Yet another duty psychiatrist reinforced the previous decision that had not been implemented, namely that if Gilbert tried to leave the ward he would be compulsorily detained. However, Gilbert again left the ward at 3.00 p.m., to the dismay of his relatives. He arrived home at 8.00 p.m. Some family members were in the house but they were unable to stop him killing his mother and then killing himself.

The critical events were characterised by poor communication within and between agencies, and by the failure of any one professional involved to 'catch and carry' the seriousness of the situation and make sure it was dealt with properly. That it happened over a weekend was no excuse. There were a number of professional staff working over the three days in question, any one of whom could have taken a more decisive responsibility. Instead, professional behaviour consisted of a series of notes and messages and inept handovers rather than a co-ordinated plan. Above all, the case illustrates the potentially fatal consequences of mishandling a mental health crisis, of not realising how quickly a situation is escalating, and of not making proper use of the formal sections of the Mental Health Act. While public concerns about care in the community have focused on a failure of the duty of care to some long-term patients discharged back into the community, this case demonstrates how those coming into the formal mental health system for the first time have equally pressing needs.

## Forensic social work

Forensic social work is social work with mentally disordered offenders. The Reed review, reporting in 1992, was commissioned by the government following a number of high profile cases in which people with mental health problems committed serious criminal offences including violent assaults. Reed recommended three main changes: the identification of mentally disordered offenders using core data jointly between all agencies involved in the process; the development of diversion schemes, so that care and treatment programmes are available to sentencers to refer into as an alternative to custody; and a range of secure and non-secure accommodation in which these programmes could be provided.[19]

Progress on implementing these recommendations has been mixed. In an overview report published in 1996, the Social Services Inspectorate found that none of the seven local authorities reviewed had tackled the fundamental issue of assembling core data about the numbers of mentally disordered offenders in their area, and their needs profiles.[20] Some agencies working together locally have decided to establish and maintain local public protection registers, which are registers of the most dangerous people known to be living in a community at any one time. Senior staff meet to share information and intelligence on a regular basis. This is the kind of initiative likely to assist in tightening up the frighteningly casual way information about potentially dangerous offenders is handled.

On the positive side, a number of court assessment schemes are in place, in which community psychiatric nurses and approved social workers cover local magistrates courts on a rota basis and screen detainees who appear to have a mental health problem. Following a large centrally funded capital programme, there are now sufficient medium-secure beds for prisoners who have been assessed as needing psychiatric care. Local authorities provide ASW cover for these beds, usually on a visiting and outreach basis. For those ASWs who work inside a medium-secure unit or high-security hospital, the stresses are huge. A key ASW role is to ensure that when patients are transferred or discharged to a community setting, that the local psychiatric team takes over the responsibility and is given full information. A key resource problem is the lack of move-on accommodation in the community for patients who need 24-hour cover. While there was a ring-fenced capital allocation to health authorities to provide more NHS beds, there was no comparable allocation to local authorities to develop move-on community services. While some have used Mental Illness Specific Grant funding to develop new services, the picture nationally is confused and inconsistent. Other community-based resources such as carers' support services are also thin on the ground.

## PEOPLE WITH PHYSICAL DISABILITIES

There are over 6 million disabled people in the UK, about 14 per cent of the population. They remain second-class citizens, with little interest being shown in them by the able-bodied majority. Good disabled access to public buildings is rare. The situation will not change much as a result of the 1995 Disability Discrimination Act, which merely encourages service providers to do what is 'reasonable' to assist disabled people to gain access to services and premises, and to promote increased employment opportunities for people with disabilities. Most employers will say that it is unreasonable for them to change because of the expense. Despite the government spending £4.5 million on raising awareness of the new legislation in 1996, 2 out of 5 employers still hadn't heard of it, and of those who had, more than half employed less than 2 disabled people.

Official attitudes show up poorly compared with the efforts made by pioneering individuals and voluntary organisations to help people with disabilities. In the early 1970s, a young paralysed man sat in his wheelchair watching a TV programme based in a Midlands hotel called *Crossroads*, in which one of the characters was disabled following an accident. It appeared to the young man that the disabled character on screen was provided with far more support than those with similar disabilities in real life, so he wrote to the producer of the series indicating the problems he and other disabled people faced. The young man's contact with the producer generated an interest and friendship. In 1974 ATV donated £10,000 for a pilot scheme to be started in Rugby. Based on the disabled young man's experience, the scheme aimed at providing respite care within the homes of people with serious disabilities or chronic diseases, thus giving the regular carer a chance to go out for a walk, go shopping or just have a rest, with the knowledge that their loved ones received the same standard of care that they themselves would normally provide. In this way, the *Crossroads* TV series gave its name to a respite care service that is now nationally recognised with over 240 schemes operating in the UK and expansion planned across Europe.

## Occupational therapy services

Occupational therapists (OTs) are professionals in their own right in a related discipline to social work. OTs often work with physiotherapists to rehabilitate people back to normal health following short-term illness or disability, i.e. a hip replacement following a fall. As with social workers, OTs are hard to recruit and retain, and there is a national shortage.

While the bulk of their work takes place with elderly people who have an age-related disability, they also assist young physically disabled people, for example road traffic accident survivors with multiple disabilities, or people who have fallen from great heights and sustained permanent spinal injuries or head injuries.

The equipment that might be provided after an OT assessment includes installing minor items such as bath rails, raised toilet seats and electric can-openers, as well as costly major adaptations to properties such as ground-floor extensions to accommodate downstairs bathrooms or extra bedrooms when a permanent disability makes climbing stairs impossible. Cash-limited budgets often mean difficult choices have to be made between spending the budget on a few major schemes or satisfying large numbers of people who need simple items of equipment. Some local authorities have stopped providing basic items such as bath and shower equipment, referring people to high street suppliers like Boots instead. That way their waiting lists look shorter. As over half of all complaints to social services are about occupational therapy service delays or lack of entitlement, managing the waiting list by administratively deleting over half of the referrals can make the authority look as if it's doing better than it really is. Local authorities may eventually set up arm's-length insurance companies of their own to ensure provision continues to be available.

Council adaptations are paid for from the local authority's housing capital programme, sometimes supplemented by social services capital or revenue funding, or by rent increases. Owner occupiers and private landlords claim Disabled Facilities Grants, which are administered either by housing or environmental services departments as part of the Renovation Grant System. Staying put, or care and repair schemes, run by housing associations, assist owner occupiers with small adaptations.

**Direct payments schemes**

Direct payments schemes have been law since 1 April 1997. A local authority has the discretion to transfer funding to a physically disabled person under 65, who can then arrange her or his own care up to an agreed sum. The funding can either be channelled directly to individuals through the care management system, or to a third party organisation able to administer the funds on behalf of disabled people.

This scheme is a direct descendant of the Independent Living Fund, set up in 1988 to do just the same. It was stopped in 1993, partly because so much money was being paid out through the benefits system to disabled people. It was replaced by a more limited fund, the Independent Living (93) Fund (ILF).

A few third party organisations grew up during the 1990s to administer funds on behalf of disabled people, partly to circumvent the law which did not allow for direct payments until 1997. The Wiltshire Independent Living Fund (WILF) was established by Wiltshire County Council and is based upon each disabled person holding a bank account in WILF's name. The disabled person is then made the authorised signatory for cheque payments. A WILF panel looks at assessments and allocates funds to individuals. WILF links strongly into a user network. The Somerset Self-Operated Care Scheme works in a similar way. Some local authorities are worried such a scheme would be hijacked by the most vocal disabled people who might not necessarily have the highest needs. This is a flawed argument. It is better to encourage vocal people to become involved, and to ensure the allocation of resources is controlled by carrying out good assessments of need.

**Rehabilitation or re-ablement services**

Medical advances are keeping people alive who only a few years ago would have died. Neo-natal intensive care baby units are keeping exceptionally premature babies alive. Before 1970, most people with severe brain injury died. Now most survive because of improved neurosurgical techniques, and the efforts of trauma teams. However, survival is often accompanied by a lasting severe disability, which requires a mixture of hospital treatment and review, and a community care package. Such services are highly expensive, on average between £10,000 and £100,000 per person per year. Rehabilitation or re-ablement services include occupational therapy, physiotherapy and social work, the different disciplines focusing on maximising the user's physical and social skills. Family members and carers will also need support, and teams of staff are usually multi-disciplinary. New trial drugs such as beta interferon may in the near future reduce the impact of conditions such as motor neurone disease and multiple sclerosis.

**Orange badge scheme**

Local authorities are responsible for administering orange badges, which are parking permits enabling people with disabilities to park in restricted zones. This is a national scheme. The mechanics of administration vary between authorities. Social services offices and libraries are often used to renew permits, which are due every three years. To be eligible for a permit, you have to be substantially and permanently disabled, confirmed by a medical recommendation. In the past, permits have been granted without question, but the criteria are now more rigorously applied and monitored for two reasons. Registering someone as disabled gives access to many services and local authorities want to gate-keep this to contain budgets. Also, the needs of orange badge users have to be weighed up against overall parking availability. A small charge, currently £2, can be collected for renewing a badge.

**PEOPLE WITH SENSORY IMPAIRMENT**

Sensory impairment can be single, either deaf or blind, partial or complete. People who are deaf and blind have dual sensory loss and are known as deafblind. Without support, people with hearing or sight impairments can become extremely isolated.

People with a sensory impairment need specialist social services in addition to general services such as information and advice, advocacy, home care, day care and supported housing which are standard requirements across social services. A care package to a deaf person might include transport to a deaf club, a minicom and a pager. A blind person might be given a braille system, possibly a braille textphone, a radio, a guide dog and a talking book. Deaf people will need an interpreting or signing service for people who use Makaton or British Sign Language, and communication services such as Typetalk (via a minicom) and the National

Telephone Relay Service. Interpreters for blind people, induction loops and deafblind communicator-guides are also available. For profoundly deafblind people, a fingerspelling interpreter may be needed. Deafblindness is more than the sum of its parts and is a disability in its own right. For instance, a minicom to use Typetalk costs about £200 for a sighted deaf person. A deafblind person needs about £5,000 of computer equipment to use the service. Often, if such expensive equipment is not provided, a person with dual sensory loss may be unnecessarily placed in residential care.

Social workers are members of specialist rehabilitation teams, who seek to maximise the sensory awareness of hearing or sight impaired people. As with the principles of dementia care, rehabilitation work in the area of sensory impairment attempts to reduce or overcome disabling effects, rather than to assume the impairment is beyond help. Specialist day care projects make use of equipment like Snoezelen rooms, which are sensory relaxation environments designed to stimulate sensory awareness.

Local authorities have to keep a register of blind and partially sighted people, and a register of those who are deaf and hard of hearing. Some authorities have established a separate deafblind register. Assessments usually follow the receipt of a BD8 form from a doctor or hospital.

**Profile of Beverley Lewis**

Beverley Lewis was 23 when she died in Gloucestershire in 1989 of neglect and starvation, weighing 3 stone 3 lbs. She had cerebral palsy, visual and hearing impairments and severe learning difficulties. She lived with her mentally ill mother, in squalid surroundings and complete isolation. The coroner concluded her death resulted from natural causes rather than lack of care, but the case aroused widespread concern. A subsequent government inspection concluded that awareness of the needs of adults with multiple disabilities was staggeringly low.[21]

Following the Lewis case, in 1992, Gloucestershire County Council established an Adults At Risk Unit. This was modelled on child protection procedures, extending to vulnerable adults the same principles of assessment, registration and multi-agency co-ordination through reviewed care plans. All referrals of adults potentially at risk of abuse or neglect from family members or other carers are investigated and assessed. Also included in at risk categories are elderly people who fall victim to systematic financial exploitation, and adults abused in institutions. In 1995–6, 255 adults were registered in Gloucestershire. The figure is rising.[22] The establishment of this service also shows how some authorities react positively to critical external inquiries and change services for the better. Other authorities carry on as before as if the critical incident meant nothing. Brent, for example, made little headway in the aftermath of the inquiry in 1986 into the death of Jasmine Beckford, a 4-year-old girl on the child protection register who was killed by her father. Multiple changes of director, demoralisation and disorganisation in the name of reorganisation meant the department was unable to change and indeed then headed off in a different direction altogether. Authorities such as Brent needed a long-term programme of continuous service improvement over many years, not a series of short-term regimes with each one starting from scratch.

## PEOPLE WITH LEARNING DIFFICULTIES

In September 1997, a French satirical weekly *Charlie-Hebdo* alleged that thousands of women with learning difficulties had been forcibly sterilised in France. The French Government promised to investigate.[23] The month before, the Junior Minister for Health, Paul Boateng, proposed a new inquiry into the actions taken by Buckinghamshire County Council in respect of the registration of residential homes run by Longcare Ltd. Criminal charges of rape, physical and mental abuse were laid against the owner Gordon Rowe, but he committed suicide before he could stand trial. His widow and other staff were convicted of lesser charges in June 1997.

People with learning difficulties are the most vulnerable adults in the adult care system, and such current allegations indicate that despite a continuous closure programme of long-stay hospitals, in which people with learning difficulties lived cut off from normal life for no reason, abuses are still continuing in new community-based settings. Often this is because the staff employed in one setting merely switch to another. Good risk assessments are needed for all people with learning difficulties, whether they are living in a long-stay institution, a residential care home, an adult fostering placement or if they are receiving a community care package.

Despite mounting evidence of continuing institutional malpractice, pressure groups such as Rescare propose that building either new village communities or core and cluster housing on the site of old long-stay hospitals, is both cost-effective and a better model of care than housing people with learning difficulties in rented supported housing in the community.[24] The debate about future provision for people with learning difficulties is one of the most lively in the social care field. Carers tend to advocate for more residential provision, while professionals support the commissioning of special needs housing and a way of life which allows maximum independence. Politicians shift uneasily between the two sides.

As a result of historical and contemporary injustices, a model of person-centred planning and care has been developed, which emphasises the rights of people with learning difficulties to an ordinary life, and one which reflects their needs at all stages. Learning disabled people are now living longer, so a needs-based service has to be designed to meet the needs of children, people of working age and older people. For some people in their fifties and sixties, planning for an ordinary life may be too little too late. A community care assessment on one man now aged 47 who had lived in long-stay residential care since he was a small child found that he did not realise you could have a cup of tea at any time of the day. He had only ever been given one at set times. He also felt unable to go out without being escorted, despite only having moderate learning difficulties and being quite able to travel limited distances. Older people with learning difficulties may prefer to live in a small unit within an old people's home, whereas young people should be given every opportunity to participate in the world of work, employment and leisure. People with high support needs and challenging behaviour may need a residential care placement, although some community-based packages can be just as effective.

A series of government inspections of services to adults with learning difficulties found that services are variable around the country, that there is a need for person-centred transport arrangements (rather than large institutional coaches ferrying people to day centres like cattle), skills teaching for front-line staff, more further education programmes, better housing and home-based support, and more employment opportunities.[25] Services in Wales are further ahead because of progress made on the All-Wales Mental Handicap (now Learning Difficulties) Strategy, which has been running since the 1980s, although repeated funding shortfalls have limited further developments.

In the last ten years, several imaginative services have been developed. Circles of support are formally established friendship groups set up so that someone with a learning difficulty has a group of people who will keep in touch with her or him. This can include relatives, workmates or friends. Advocacy schemes uphold the rights of people with learning difficulties in all situations in which they find themselves. Supported employment schemes find work for people with moderate learning difficulties with caring employers, and the largest public and private sector employers have responded. Some projects are funded on a Europe-wide basis. The CISSTA (Coping with sexuality: support and training at work) project, set up to support women with learning difficulties cope with their sexuality (and that of others) in the workplace, has attracted European Social Fund money for three years from 1998–9, and links projects in Havering, North East London, with similar projects in Southern Ireland, Rome and Sweden, the purpose being to promote a Europe-wide approach to supported employment. Drama projects for people with learning difficulties can become semi-professional. Some students join Equity and pursue acting careers.

Another way of supporting people in the community is through support tenants living near to or with the person needing support. Support tenants live rent-free in exchange for providing about ten hours' care per week, and of course being available at night and over the weekend if something goes wrong. In a housing development of ten special needs flats, one or two can be made available for support tenants. Support tenants need to be vetted and recruited against an explicit brief of what type of support is required. Expectations have to be made clear so there are no misunderstandings.

Live-in volunteers are a model of supporting people with 24-hour-a-day support needs. Organisations like Community Service Volunteers have run such schemes for over twenty years. Two volunteers may live with the person needing support, on a shift basis, working normal 35-hour weeks. The following profile shows the benefits of such a scheme.

**Profile of Irma**

Irma lives in a four-bedroom house in North London. She is 37 years old. She shares a tenancy with another woman who is about to move in, and two CSVs who have a bedroom each in the house and support both Irma and her co-tenant. The landlord is a housing association with lengthy experience of developing social housing schemes, although Irma lives in a Victorian terraced house and not a special needs housing development.

Irma has severe learning difficulties and a number of physical disabilities such as arthritis in her arms, epilepsy and partial sightedness. She grew up in the West Indian island of Dominica and lived with her grandmother as a child. In her late twenties she came to England to live with her mother, but their relationship became strained, possibly because of the long period of absence or possibly because her mother found Irma's support needs were too high.

Irma was placed initially in a private residential care home, which she remembers as a troubled experience, because of the aggression shown towards her by another resident. From there she moved to a small group home for four women with learning difficulties, run by Hackney Independent Living Team, a specialist independent sector provider. This was better for Irma, but she still found living in a group put her under great pressure. She craved a home of her own. A risk assessment was carried out, with a care plan that would guarantee Irma enough support to be safe in the community but living a much more ordinary life. Ordinary living, for people living in institutional care, is a basic but ultimate goal.

This is the first time Irma has owned anything of her own. She is proud of her possessions, referring to them as 'my taps', 'my hot water', 'my toaster', 'my kettle'. She is supported by her outreach worker, Ruth, who has known Irma for over 6 years, and her 2 CSVs, Clair and Kirsten. Clair and Kirsten are graduates of psychology and biochemistry respectively, and are in their early twenties, living with Irma for a year before developing their careers. When they move on, it is planned that other CSVs will move in, although they will move out in a phased way so Irma always has someone in her house she knows well. CSVs are paid £51 a week plus expenses for a 35-hour working week plus night shift cover. They are assessed for suitability, and then matched with a particular situation. In fact, Irma carries out most personal care herself, and Clair and Kirsten are really there just to support her and communicate with her. Irma's highest support need is the need for constant communication. In the past she has been labelled as autistic, which in her case seems to have meant high communication needs, but not an inability to communicate at all.

She works for three days a week washing up in a staff canteen for office workers run as a café project to train people with learning difficulties up to National Vocational Qualification Level 1. Takings are apparently booming. Irma enjoys her job immensely, more than the day centre she attends for the other two days of the working week. She is taken to and from work and the day centre by Dial-a-Ride, a transport service for people with disabilities. She goes to church on Sundays, for which she is receiving travel training from a member of the local sensory impairment team, to help her recognise a safe route. Her partial sightedness restricts her vision to bright colours and broad outlines.

Her care package costs about £500 per week. Her previous residential care placement cost £733 per week. Her house was furnished using a community care grant from the Benefits Agency and grants from charities. Net of paying rent and other expenses, Irma has £81 a week to spend on food, clothes and other items she chooses. In residential care she had £13.65 money to spend, which is the standard personal allowance for anyone living in residential care. She is better off financially as well as psychologically.

She has just found a more sensitive GP who is reducing her levels of phenobarbitone, which she has taken for years to control her epilepsy. She has not had a fit for some years, so her GP is looking carefully at establishing her on the right dose, which makes a change from her previous GP who merely wrote out endless repeat prescriptions. This illustrates how vital it is for people with learning difficulties to have good access to primary health care.

Each community in Britain has a view about reprovision programmes for people with learning difficulties. While it is fashionable for social services staff to brush off  local opposition to new community care resettlement hostels as NIMBY (not in my back yard) prejudice, it is important to understand the concerns and rights of neighbours. Neighbours need to know there is someone in authority they can turn to if they are concerned about noise levels, threatening behaviour, or if they are worried that a service user needs more care or monitoring. They need to know that if they make complaints or express anxieties, these will be followed up rather than ridiculed or ignored. They also need to know that if there are major problems in a resettlement unit, staff will take decisive action. If the responsible authority handles community concerns positively, professional values rarely need to be sacrificed, and more often than not projects settle down inside a neighbourhood.

Nationally, a start has been made to put in place long-term community services. In 1996, the government committed £154 million to the Supported Employment Service, which finds work for people with disabilities. That sum had increased by 16 per cent since 1991.

E-mail is popular with people with learning difficulties, as they can control the pace of conversation in a way that is sometimes difficult with face-to-face speech. Some Internet sites are highly accessible to people with learning difficulties. For example, Northamptonshire People First organisation is trying to establish a Europe-wide People First over the Internet.

## PEOPLE WITH HIV/AIDS

People who are HIV positive or who develop AIDS have long-term health and social care needs. Responsibilities for their care are usually shared between health authorities and social services. Services can either be residential, in hospital units, to treat infections or to give treatments, or in hospices, to be cared for while dying, especially in the absence of family carers or friends. Most services, however, are community-based. Typical community services include volunteer support projects, drop-in services such as café projects, community nursing, advice lines, counselling, and information projects such as the *National Aids Manual* which gives information on all available treatments. Many services are the same services you find in place for any disadvantaged group, like advocacy services, welfare rights advice and information, housing and legal advice, home care, and child care support for parents with HIV/AIDS. Social services has been funded to provide these services through the AIDS support grant (ASG), and most of the money is spent on small voluntary sector contracts. As with a number of other specific grants, the government pays 70 per cent of the cost up to the allowed level, and the local authority has to contribute 30 per cent. If it doesn't pay its 30 per cent, it loses the 70 per cent, and some local authorities have not claimed their ASG because of not feeling able to commit the 30 per cent. The government repeatedly warns it may end the ASG and expect local authorities to fund HIV/AIDS services through mainstream funding.

There is a strong tradition of user involvement in the development and running of services. Many culturally specific services have been set up to support sufferers in ethnic minority communities, particularly African communities. Same race outreach development workers have opened up HIV issues in particular communities, contacting people via garages, hairdressers and other businesses owned by people from the same race and culture.

Nobody with AIDS survives. Everyone dies eventually, although new combination drug therapies slow the process down considerably and may offer hope of preventing the HIV virus developing into AIDS. The motto for services could be to promote both quality of life and quality of death. Because people with AIDS are terminally ill, working in this area is highly stressful.

In the UK, a disproportionately high number of gay men and bisexual men are affected, although there is a growing rate of infection among heterosexuals, and more cases notified of children infected, nine out of ten through mother to child transmission. Exposure categories differ in different parts of the UK. In Scotland one in three people affected are injecting drug users, whereas in the rest of the UK it is one in twenty-five.

That apart, the trends are changing quickly, and the percentage of those infected who are injecting drug users in Scotland is now falling. Health promotion work in the HIV/AIDS field is often dazzling and exciting. For years it has been the trendiest cause to back. Practitioners working with people dying from AIDS who are ostracised within society are often angered by the razzamatazz of concerts, roadshows and fun runs, which seem to glamorise an extremely ugly disease. Nevertheless, prevention is the most important service of all, and people changing to a safer lifestyle by ceasing to have unprotected sex and using safer drug-injecting methods, would save more lives than treatment programmes ever can. The Health Education Authority's Internet website, which features animated graphic images and full information, was voted one of the most popular websites in 1995 with over 200,000 visitors.[26] The publicity has also helped groups to fund-raise and the potential ending of the Aids Support Grant means continued publicity such as launches and dramatic events might be the only way of maintaining decent levels of service in the future. Public figures have always supported charities, and their support is invaluable in terms of helping directly or indirectly with fund-raising, and keeping issues in front of the public that otherwise would scarcely be mentioned at all.

### Profile of Nigel

Nigel is a long-term survivor of AIDS. For how long to come, he doesn't know. He is currently taking new combination drugs as part of a controlled trial, and is feeling better and better. Previously a banqueting chef, Nigel came out in 1985 and met his partner Alistair in 1986. In 1990, after his partner was diagnosed as HIV positive, Nigel too was diagnosed positive, following chest infections and strange rashes appearing on the inside of his legs. For six months, he denied the diagnosis, and pretended it wasn't happening. Alistair died in 1992. It was around that time that Nigel got involved with social services. Alistair was receiving an intensive home care service in his last months, and the help of a specialist care manager from the local HIV/AIDS social work team, Liz, who is effectively an advocate and friend, first to Alistair and now to Nigel in his own right. Liz is also a qualified occupational therapist and makes sure Nigel has the right equipment and adaptations at home to maintain his independence. She also sorts out any difficulties with benefits he has. In the same way, Kim, the home care worker, now supports Nigel, having originally helped Alistair. Kim has given Nigel her home phone number and mobile phone number even though it's against the rules, and she's available to him round the clock. For Nigel, there is no weak link in the professional chain. Even his housing association is helpful and he has medical cover from a specialist unit at a local hospital, from a clinical nurse specialist and from a community physiotherapist who visits weekly. He receives a genuinely seamless inter-agency service.

## PEOPLE WHO MISUSE DRUGS

It is in the field of HIV/AIDS and substance misuse – misuse of drugs, alcohol and other solutions like glue and other solvents – that the mixed economy of care is thriving. The voluntary sector is leading the way in provision, with local authorities very much the funders and commissioners of community support services.

Although there are some specialist health-run drug dependency
units, and rehabilitation units, private and voluntary sector rehab
projects are well established, many of them having been set up when
the casualties of the 1960s' and 1970s' drug scenes began to emerge
as a social group.

A small amount of government money is available in the form of
the Drugs and Alcohol Specific Grant, and is only available for
voluntary sector schemes. In 1997–8, priority is being given to
projects which help homeless people with a drug problem. Grants
are made on the basis of outcome funding, where the applicants
clearly set out how the project will help drug misusers via 'customer
milestones'. Positive outcomes are hard to specify because of the
built-in certainty that a high number of drug misusers will relapse.
It is not possible to tell in advance who can be helped to stop taking
hard drugs, and who can't. This makes all social services work with
drug misusers something of a lottery. In order to offer effective
help, assessors have to respond quickly as soon as the user asks for
help. Any delay and she or he will probably move on quickly out of
reach. A lot of money is wasted on people who go into rehab
projects and fail. Rehabilitation projects use a variety of treatment
models, some British and some American. All involve both physical
and psychological help. The drug treatment world has its crusaders,
who are almost evangelical about their own 'product'. In general,
however, drugs workers are hard and seasoned professionals who
take the view that, when asked for, treatment should be made available to all who ask because even in the fourth or fifth attempt at
rehab, an addict might be helped to come off drugs. Local authorities and health authorities sometimes have hard choices to make, as
to whether to repeatedly fund a hard drugs user through expensive
rehabilitation programmes, when those funds could be used for a
range of preventative schemes. The UK is not yet like certain
American states, where the public vote by referendum for which
treatments should be freely available. In the UK, choices are made
behind closed doors. As part of the Task Force to Review Services
to Drug Misusers, the National Treatment Outcome Research Study
is tracking 1,100 drug misusers who started treatment in 1995
through the major treatment and care programmes until the year
2001. Its first findings, published in 1997, showed marked improvements in key problem behaviours following treatment. These
improvements had been maintained whether or not the programme
was mandatory or voluntary.[27] This finding contrasts with the

general public perception, sometimes police-fuelled, that drug-taking in the UK is out of control. There are many aspects of health and social care, such as the treatment of mental illness, where we now know more about how it is caused and how to treat it more successfully. But as professional health and social care agencies become objectively more successful, so the public attitude towards their work seems to become more hostile.

At the official level, anti-drugs services are co-ordinated through drug action teams, set up in 1995 following the 'Tackling Drugs Together' initiative.[28] This has attempted to bring together all government departments in a single co-ordinated initiative. Local authorities and health authorities were required to set up drug action teams and produce a work programme showing how they were tackling drug-related problems at the local level. Work programmes include enforcement programmes to curb drug dealers, treatment programmes, harm reduction services to assist drug misusers, and drugs prevention work, particularly aimed at schools, through drugs education sessions, and young people, through publicity and outreach work. These programmes are often delivered and co-ordinated through community drugs teams. The role of GPs in shared care arrangements is important, and many projects support, train and develop GPs in providing 'optimum' patient care.

Solving the drugs problem is impossible, because of elusive supply routes to an expectant market. Within each average local authority area of a quarter of a million people, the drug economy can be worth up to £400 million a year, making illicit drug supply often the most common form of local employment. Users also purchase in a complex way. A number of methadone users supplement their treatment with freely available street heroin. The price of heroin on the streets in UK cities has remained fairly stable over the last fifteen years, and supplies of hard drugs like heroin and crack cocaine are holding up better than supplies of soft drugs like cannabis, despite intensive efforts by customs and excise officers, regional drugs squads, and the National Criminal Intelligence Service to seize new supplies. Stockpiles are being held in Europe and the Single Market offers greater scope for smugglers. Drug-related crime is rampant and hard to tackle. For instance, 50 per cent of adults formally supervised by the Inner London Probation Service are known to be drug misusers. Prisoners are more likely to use heroin than cannabis because it passes through the body quicker and is less likely to show up in a routine urine test. Drugs are so freely available in British prisons and cheaper than on the outside that a prison sentence can easily lead to drug dependency. Harm reduction is therefore a more realistic as well as a safer policy. Harm reduction schemes include needle exchange schemes to prevent infection through the use of shared or dirty needles; drugs advice and information projects; arrest referral schemes in which support and counselling are offered to people arrested for a drug-related crime – to be effective these have to be available at the time of arrest, not weeks afterwards; peer education programmes, where ex-users advise young people about the dangers of drugs; and 'safe dancing' projects in clubs and raves, in which drugs workers circulate on the floor to advise young people directly about the dangers of taking the sorts of recreational drugs like ecstasy that are freely available to young people who go clubbing.

Anti-drugs education programmes are now well embedded in the UK. For example, within the 147 Football Association Centres of Excellence for over 10,000 9–16 year olds, there is an awareness and education programme. Positive tests of professional footballers fell from 12 to 5 between the 1993–4 and the 1996–7 seasons.

## PEOPLE WHO MISUSE ALCOHOL

While drug misuse creates more headlines, alcohol misuse is just as big a problem in Britain. Alcohol abuse is commonly associated with child abuse, domestic violence and mental illness. According to the National Disabilities Commission, alcohol is involved in up to 40 per cent of domestic violence and 30 per cent of child protection cases. It is now usually separated from drug misuse and viewed as a social problem in its own right, whereas until recently in professional circles it was the junior partner of drug misuse within the umbrella concept of 'substance misuse'. Substance misuse also includes misuse of solvents or any other substances.

It is common to think of drugs as providing the quickest route either to nirvana or to an altered state of mind. Alcohol, drunk to excess, can do the same, and is much more freely available. It can also be more dangerous. Alcohol drunk to excess can damage virtually all the growing cells in the body of a foetus, which is more harmful in the longer-term than being born addicted to heroin because of transmission through the body of the mother. It is of course not illegal to drink yourself into a stupor, and, until recent public information campaigns took up the theme of the wider dangers of alcohol, heavy drinking has been regarded as nearly normal and quite British. It is only relatively recently that the moral majority in the UK has begun to realise that lager louts and drink-related violence are simply extreme forms of an approved habit. Much the same has happened with smokers, who are now well on the way to being regarded as a lesser species by the moral majority. The 1990s' lifestyle panics about BSE come at the same time as renewed campaigns for the legalisation of cannabis. This is the ultimate triumph of the 1960s' pot-smoking vegetarian generation.

While there may be a widespread and growing awareness of the risks to young people associated with teenage drinking, especially mixing drink and drugs, this seems to have had little impact so far on teenage lifestyles. Adolescent drunk driving convictions are on the increase, and many incidents involve crashes and severe personal injury. Teenage smoking is on the increase for similar reasons. The more adults frown upon it, the more exciting it is. We find it hard in the UK to be objective about alcohol. The concern in the mid-1990s about the sale of alcopops to teenagers may be misplaced. Objectively, alcopops might be far less dangerous to young people than beer or spirits.

Care management for problem drinkers can involve referral to a detoxification (detox) unit, or to a wet centre, in which drink is available but only as part of a counselling and therapy package. Otherwise, most detox units ban drinking just as most drug rehab units ban drug-taking, or seek to. Alcohol abuse can be difficult to detect, even when it is chronic and severe.

As with any other community care service, the most important elements are awareness and prevention. Alcohol Concern and other alcohol advisory services prefer to intervene before major problems occur, offering advice and counselling services to anyone worried about their own drinking pattern or a close relative or friend's drinking. They use a number of techniques to help control problem drinking, such as drink diaries in which the drinker faithfully records every drink they have. This aims to confront the high level of denial shown by many drinkers, who kid themselves and others they are not really drinking that much.

Alcoholism is a desperate social and medical condition. Several drug treatments are available such as Disulfiram, or 'antabuse', which induces a thoroughly unpleasant reaction and even unconsciousness if you have a drink while taking it. It was originally developed as a treatment for stomach worms, and its deterrent effect works best if it is part of a wider treatment programme including counselling. Alcoholics also need high levels of personal support in order to stay dry. One of the main characters in the BBC soap opera, *Eastenders*, Phil Mitchell, became an alcoholic and the producers were widely praised for showing a mass audience the sordid and sad reality of alcoholism, demonstrating how difficult it is to kick the habit once it has been formed. The episodes show how the media in the UK can contribute to greater social awareness without sacrificing dramatic appeal.

## SERVICES TO CARERS

It is easy to over-estimate the amount of help given by social services. While some people receive intensive help, and the general level of support for people in need of community care services has increased with the community care reforms, the vast majority of care is provided by close family members, unsupported and unrecognised in what they are doing. In 1994, there were an estimated seven million carers in the UK, according to the Carers National Association and the Princess Royal Trust for Carers.[29] A quarter are involved in care in the home for many hours in the week. Nearly two million carers provide more than 20 hours' care a week: 1 in 5 carers look after more than one person. The average time spent caring is eleven years. Carers may be saving the government over £30 billion a year.[30] They only ask for help when they reach breaking point.

Official carers differ from unofficial carers. Official carers, like foster carers or paid volunteers, are often recruited by word of mouth and personal contact, and there are many tribes of carers – carers of children with disabilities where the vocation of caring is inter-generational, with children and even grandchildren following suit, and other groups of carers formed through contact at churches and other social clubs. Unofficial carers are family members and neighbours who take on a caring role for a specific person and do not go beyond that.

Technically, unofficial carers can ask for an assessment of their own needs, and this basic right is set out in the Carers (Recognition and Services) Act, which became law in April 1996. The Carers National Association, in a survey of the first year of implementation of the Act, found that only 18 per cent of carers had asked for an assessment, although 59 per cent of those assessed were happy with the outcome.[31] Services cannot be provided to the carer directly, but services for the person being looked after can be provided. The spirit of the legislation implied that the state would take over some of the care from the carer, enabling the carer to carry on longer or simply to be given a break at times. The recognition element should not be overlooked as that is sufficient for many carers, as long as they have someone in officialdom to turn to if they are desperate.

Carers and local authorities have an uneasy relationship, as both are in many ways dependent upon the other. Rather than working together, they often see themselves as mutually exclusive. Little has changed since the new legislation and the movement for carers' rights has not been advanced that far. Carers are reluctant to ask for help, and local authorities tend to assume carers are OK until they tell them otherwise. Carers are the last people to scream, but they do suffer from above-average levels of loneliness, depression and loss of income. Carers often have to give up work because of a lack of flexible working schemes.

The big questions many carers want to ask can't be answered straightforwardly. Many are concerned for the future of the person they're caring for if they, the carer, were to fall under a bus. Local authorities tell them they will assess the person needing care at the time and take it from there. This is all too vague for carers, who want to hear that something definite has been planned. Communication difficulties and mistrust between local authorities and local carers can be reduced by the appointment of a carers' co-ordinator, or assigning responsibility for carer liaison to a named member of staff whose job it is to build up confidence between carers and social services staff. Even better, but still rare, are independently funded carers' centres, which can advocate and lobby on behalf of local carers.

# Chapter 6

# Whose service is it, anyway?
## Involving service users

## USER EMPOWERMENT

The replacement of the description 'client' with 'service user' in the 1980s was more than a change of terminology. 'User empowerment', 'user-centred services', 'user participation' were some of the most frequently used terms that peppered conference papers, journal articles, government and other reports and pronouncements. 'User empowerment' was, perhaps, the decade's Big Idea and one which perhaps because it was employed with a certain lack of precision drew together the political right and left, professionals and service users, and the statutory and voluntary sectors. As everyone was against sin, no-one would doubt the conventional wisdom that users had a part to play in the shaping of service provision. But when that commitment was more honoured in rhetoric than in practice, it was exactly *how* it was to be implemented which caused debate. Where were the lines to be drawn? What did 'involvement' mean? 'Involvement', 'empowerment' and 'participation' were frequently used interchangeably, something which contributed to the general lack of definition which itself gave rise to frequent misunderstandings between users and local authorities about how the latter saw the former and vice versa.

User empowerment is the end of which involvement is the means. Empowerment recognises strengths rather than weaknesses. This is important for social workers: being negative can make users of services feel powerless and depressed. At the root of empowerment are attempts to help users move away from a dependency culture, whether it is dependency on state support or defeatism about a personal situation.

The Griffiths Report (1988) made no mention of social work.

The NHS and Community Care Act 1990, which Griffiths spawned, appeared to threaten social work with the new care management, for which nurses, teachers, occupational therapists and domiciliary care organisers seemed as well fitted. But by contrast, the White Paper, *Caring for People: Community Care in the Next Decade and Beyond* (Department of Health 1989), which had preceded the legislation, had stated that the coming legislative changes were 'designed to give people a greater say in how they live their lives and the services they need to help them to do so'. A statement, which followed the White Paper, by William Waldegrave, then Health Secretary, was also unequivocal in its intentions: 'We must be on the side of the user rather than the provider, to ensure that services are provided efficiently with emphasis on quality.' He went on to refer to 'management systems powered by the voice of the user' (quoted in Philpot 1994b).

This seemed to set service users' voices and status, not just their needs, firmly at the centre. This was given further official sanction when the guidance from the Social Services Inspectorate of the Department of Health, which followed the Act, was published in 1991. This stated, equally trenchantly: 'The whole rationale for this reorganisation is the empowerment of users and carers' (Social Services Inspectorate 1991).

Such official attitudes need to be contrasted with earlier vaguer, less formal expressions of support for service users. For example, in 1968, the Seebohm Report had given support to what it termed 'citizen participation' (Committee on Local Authority and Allied Personal Social Services 1968). It recommended the participation of individuals and groups in service provision. However, while this encouragement was welcome and very much within the ethos of its time (as 'participation' was also a buzz word in other areas like local authority environmental planning), it made no great impact in the way the new social services departments conducted themselves with regard to those with whom they worked. In 1982 the Barclay Report was produced by a committee set up by the then Department of Health and Social Security, but the committee distanced itself from the department in that it operated under the aegis of the National Institute for Social Work. The report referred to 'clients, relations, neighbours and volunteers [who] become partners with the social worker in developing and providing social care networks'. It also later stated that 'an attempt must be made to see people and their needs as a whole and to take account of their view about what services, if any, are provided'. Barclay reaffirmed Seebohm's belief in community-oriented provision. Although Barclay foreshadowed the later interest in informal caring in the community, the report was safely shelved after polite ministerial words.

The White Paper, *Caring for People*, while leaning heavily on Griffiths' recommendations, placed great emphasis on the creation of internal markets and the financial and management arrangements consequent upon the reforms, at the expense of informal carers and neighbourhood networks, as did the succeeding NHS and Community Care Act. The intention of the reforms was, according to the government, to increase choice for those who used services. Thus, users came to be regarded, in theory and rhetoric at least, as centre stage: their needs were to be served, not the needs of those supplying services. If social workers and their managers looked behind the rhetoric they could see a major conceptual change. Adams (1996) dates the mid-1970s as the period when 'confidence among professionals in the rehabilitative and improving power of individual treatment was beginning to run low'. Thus, gradually, the change that took place was from one of models of 'treatment' of a 'client' to one of 'empowerment' of a 'user'.

Adams calls this the 'democratic approach'. However, while it may give professionals a warm feeling of solidarity with those with whom they work, it overlooks the fact that – with regard to social workers who possess statutory powers of intervention, such as approved social workers in mental health and child protection workers – the interests of professional and user do not always coincide. Indeed, they may at times be diametrically opposed – the parent of the child who is to be taken into care, the person with mental health problems who is to be sectioned (compulsorily detained) under the Mental Health Act. In what sense can users be 'empowered' under these circumstances? True, the parent can be assisted to resist the care proceedings if they think them unjust; the person with mental health problems can be assisted to oppose sectioning. But by whom? Not the social worker who instigates the proceedings. Such assistance and advocacy can only come from a third party – a voluntary agency, a self-advocacy group, a civil rights agency or a citizen advocate.

The impression can sometimes be given by social workers that they are on the users' side, that the dilemmas of their roles as social police officers, as representatives of a public agency, as holders of coercive (if necessary) statutory powers cannot only be smoothed over but do not actually exist. Beresford (1994) makes the point when he writes:

One of the paradoxes of [in this case mental health] legislation is that it gives people powers and responsibilities who are ambivalent about exercising them and because of this it is all too easy to become oblivious to the real struggles of someone from a personal and social point of view.

But it is also the case that users have not only criticised the way social workers have exercised their controlling powers. They have also criticised their behaviour when its intention has been to offer support. Ellis (1993) found this in her study of the participation of carers and users of services in assessment. She refers to 'differential power' between participants which influences how needs are defined. Too often the worker undertaking the assessment brought to the process his or her own value judgements whether users were 'deserving' or 'undeserving', whether the provision of services might make them dependent, or they had their own ideas about what the user needed. For example, Ellis gives the case of an elderly woman, fearful and isolated due to sight loss, who wanted someone to take her out occasionally, especially for shopping. Yet she was seen by the social worker as suffering 'a hierarchy of losses' in which 'the traumatic loss of a parent was the most fundamental and unresolved issue', while sight loss was the least significant.

While some commentators such as Croft and Beresford (1996) see the conceptual change as one led by users themselves, in their agitation through the user led groups they have formed, this is only partly true. It would be unjust to the social work profession not to recognise its own role in this: in the late 1970s, for example, the British Association of Social Workers was talking about the social worker as 'an enabler' – someone who was assisting the 'client' away from dependence and towards independence.

Enabling, however, is not empowerment. Empowerment is a shift of power from professional to user and enhances the individual's position in relation to authority, however represented (by the state, local authority, professional). But notions like enabling were glimmering embryonic forms of what was to come. It is possible to see Biestek's principles of casework (Biestek 1961) as consistent with ideas of encouraging empowerment. The principles which would especially apply would be those of a non-judgemental attitude and acceptance on the part of the social worker; 'individualisation' (recognising the personal individuality of the client no matter to which group – female, black, poor, disabled – they belong); and client self-determination, even if Biestek saw the 'relationship' as the 'dynamic interaction of attitudes and emotions between the caseworker and the client, with the purpose of helping the client achieve a better adjustment between himself and his environment', a purpose which would not be endorsed by radical social workers or many services users. It is also worth noting that social work is one of the few professions which tends to talk about disempowering itself, and sometimes acts to do so rather than accruing power to itself.

## A TRUE CHOICE?

Another example of a social work method where, arguably, users can have a direct impact on practice is in task-centred social work. This focuses on solving problems which the user thinks important through the completion of small tasks. In his description of the task-centred method, Marsh (1996) says two principles arise from the observation that users often face enormous difficulties and pressures in meeting the problems of their daily life and tackle them by feats of ingenuity usually unknown to the practitioner. Thus, task-centred social work recognises, first, that users have a great deal of expertise in coping with their circumstances and, second, that they understand their circumstances better than can professionals. Marsh comments:

> Task-centred social work is based on users' strengths. It is those strengths which will provide change, sometimes in  directions that users clearly wanted, sometimes in directions they have agreed to, however reluctantly, as a result of legal  processes. Tasks use those strengths and fill in any gaps in  strengths.

Today, user empowerment (or involvement) tends to be seen much more in terms of the way social services is organised and provided than in which social work approach is best suited to the user. But the so-called revolution has only gone so far. Croft and Beresford (1996) sum up by saying:

> The indications from both service users and independent research findings is [sic] that user involvement [in formal consultative

structures concerned with bureaucratic and administrative functions] has been patchy and qualified, and its gains limited. . . . Service users have more often experienced user involvement as stressful, diversionary and unproductive.

It has been bedevilled by a failure of all those involved in social services – practitioners, managers, users, politicians and carers – to agree on a working definition of user involvement. One set of definitions has been expressed as follows (Philpot 1994b):

Involvement is a blanket term which covers all sorts of activities, from membership of planning groups of users to training staff and running services.

Participation has a precise meaning – taking part in decision making – but, through frequent use, has come to have the same general meaning as involvement.

Empowerment is often linked to user involvement. Managers cannot give power to service users, even through giving funding, but they can help to create an enabling environment in which users can do things for themselves.

Too often user involvement is something which is seen as an add-on, or it is confused with consultation with users. However, if it is to have a real meaning, if it is to be a reality in service provision and planning, it is something which has to permeate the whole organisation: its tenor, attitudes, policies and practices. A key element of this is in staff training. Parsloe and Stevenson (1993) (looking at practice in this area across a number of social services departments) and Marsh and Fisher (1992) (looking at services for children in Bradford and Westminster) said that training people in an atmosphere which, while not unsympathetic to user involvement, has itself not absorbed its underlying principles and values, is to sow seed on stony ground. Parsloe and Stevenson define empowerment as 'both a process and a goal'. But what can this mean in practice? Philpot (1994b) defines a continuum of examples from minimum to maximum involvement. This is shown in Table 6.1.

Thus, the theory of user involvement has been worked out (even allowing for a confusion over terms), and the idea is accepted but the practice is lacking. In part this is due to the fact that the high expectations raised by the community care legislation have been disappointed. Services led by the needs of users and assessments based on the needs of those assessed (which were the stated aims of

*Table 6.1*  Continuum of examples from minimum to maximum involvement

| Degree of involvement | Type | Explanation |
| --- | --- | --- |
| Minimum | Information | Users are given information about developments through talks, newsletters or leaflets. |
| | Consultation | A variety of means (surveys, stakeholder conferences, smaller meetings) are used to elicit user views which will be taken into consideration when decisions are made. |
| | Partnership | Managers, professionals and users work together to plan and reach decisions about the service. |
| Maximum | User control | Budgets may be delegated to users to run their own services or carry out work on behalf of commissioning agencies, e.g. quality monitoring. |

the reforms) have given way, in a climate of financial stringency, to services determined by available resources, with assessment criteria being drawn tighter and tighter.

It is also the case that choice – another defining term of the community care changes – has been found in many places to be a chimera: users do not, for the most part, have choice in the services which are on offer.

Even in the drawing up of community care plans, user involvement has been found to be the exception rather than the rule. Local authorities are required, by law, to draw up these plans which set out the needs of the local population and how they are to be met. They are often very detailed documents, not merely vague statements of intent. Government guidance and the legislation itself make it incumbent upon local authorities to consult with health and housing agencies, voluntary organisations, private agencies and user and carer groups. However, no specific guidance is given as to the form which this consultation should take or the means by which it will be carried out. A study by Glendinning and Bewley (1992) of ninety-nine of the plans showed that local authorities had used the existing joint planning arrangements with the NHS and that there was extensive consultation with the voluntary sector. However, only 16 per cent of the plans stated clearly that user groups had been consulted in the planning process, and, where they had been, this was usually only at the level of working groups. The authors stated that

> while extensive and creative attempts have been made to publicise the plans, particularly in their draft and final stages, less attention seems to have been directed to ensuring that disabled people, whether as service users or local residents, are actively involved in the actual planning process itself.

Later and more detailed studies (Hoyes and Lart 1992; and Martin and Gaster 1993) have confirmed these findings.

In another study by Hoyes and Lart  (Hoyes *et al.* 1993), users' views of what happened are recorded. Comments quoted include: 'The current community care plan doesn't reflect the consultations'; 'The drafts aren't readable for most people'; 'They have consulted but are the services stitched up already?'

But while practitioners and local authorities can be seen to be lacking in a practical attachment to participation, it is also the case that government and the courts have been unhelpful. For example, in 1992 (only a year after the Social Services Inspectorate's guidance quoted above), the High Court ruled that residents of local authority elderly persons' homes had no right to be consulted before decisions were made to close the homes.

## SELF-ADVOCACY AND NORMALISATION

Booth (1996) argues that 'it is inconceivable' that the goals of participation can be met without vigorous self-advocacy and citizen advocacy movements. Self-advocacy is where groups of users – most commonly people with mental health problems and people with a learning difficulty – band together to speak on their own behalf, defend their rights and organise in their own interests. Citizen advocacy is where representatives of people who are unable to speak for themselves are chosen and undertake to speak for those who cannot. Sections 1–3 of the Disabled Persons (Representation) Act 1986 gave users the statutory right to have a citizen advocate if they wished for one. The then Health Minister (and later Secretary of State for Health) Virginia Bottomley refused to implement the Act claiming that forthcoming community care legislation would bring about the same aims, when, in fact, that Act contained no such provision. While citizen advocacy is widespread, it remains something which is accepted only at the discretion of health trusts and social services departments against whom, of course, citizen advocates may have to take action.

Self-advocacy is a practical example of empowerment. Since 1980 many groups comprising users of social services have grown up, often because of disenchantment with services and perceived injustice at the hands of professionals. Among these are PAIN (Parents Against Injustice) for parents who have been investigated on suspicion of abusing their children, without, it is alleged, just cause. Survivors Speak Out was founded in 1986 by those who had been through the mental health system, often as patients in hospitals, who have always been stigmatised and often damaged by the experience. Physically disabled people have also revolted against statutory services and come together in groups like the British Council of Disabled People. There are also user-led groups for people with learning difficulties (People First) and young people in care (National Voice).

Physically disabled people argue that their disability is socially constructed – a common thread among user self-help groups is to attack 'medical models' of disability – through problems of physical access and social discrimination. So far as the provision of services is concerned, physically disabled people have been in the forefront of the (successful) campaign to allow 'direct payments'. Until the Community Care (Direct Payments) Act 1996 local authorities were not permitted by law to make direct payments to users of services so that they could themselves purchase services. (There were ways around some of the problems but these involved constructing byzantine systems to allow payments to be made to third party agencies.) Legislation now makes this possible. The ability to receive payment to purchase a service (and helpers) of one's own choice is a very significant shift of power from professional to user, from local authority to individual. It is also another interesting example of where the philosophies of a Conservative Government coincided with a radical view of welfare held by those who were not the natural allies of the Conservative Party.

Direct payments are also one way of meeting the inherent problems identified in the concept of 'normalisation'. This idea was developed in Scandinavia and in the USA and emphasises the desirability of people with a learning difficulty living lives as normal as possible through the provision of proper jobs, ordinary housing and access to non-segregated leisure pursuits. It is 'a statement about how services can reflect the basic rights of people with learning difficulties in an egalitarian society' (Emerson 1992). It was further developed, in the learning difficulties field, by Wolfensberger (Wolfensberger and Thomas 1983) who put forward the concept of 'social role valorisation' – that is, that normalisation should be concerned with the way people with learning difficulties (though the idea was transferable to other groups of service users) were perceived and portrayed socially and that they should have 'socially valued' roles in the community. An improvement in their social image and competence would change social perceptions of them and would thus lead to their being able to live ordinary and valued lives. Behind this idea is that of self-determination and behind self-determination is self-advocacy. But some critics like Chappell (1992) have seen problems with this:

> Normalisation offers a theory of how to improve services. As services are controlled by professionals, normalisation has enabled professionals to retain a key role in the debate about quality. It does not challenge the legitimacy of the professional role in the lives of people with learning difficulties. It has enabled professionals to adapt to deinstitutionalisation by developing new models of practice. It therefore continues to legitimise authority.

Much has been written about how the closure of long-stay hospitals ('deinstitutionalisation') has not led to the provision of ordinary living but mini-institutions through hostel-like accommodation (Collins 1995). It would be difficult to see how direct payments, which apply to local authorities and not NHS trusts, which ran the old institutions and their successors, would solve this problem. However, housing is not the only need of people with a learning difficulty (albeit an important one) and increasingly people with learning difficulties will come within the ambit of local authorities, not NHS trusts (because so many now have never experienced the old institutional care). For them direct payments can make some impact on the problems to which Chappell draws attention.

## CONCLUSIONS

Grand statements about users' interests predominating over those of professionals will be hollow unless those interests are given practical effect in the way services are shaped and provided. Not only do research and experience indicate that there is a long way to go but there is nothing in the policies and proposals of the Labour Government that marks it out as different from its Conservative predecessor in this regard. It is arguable that the government will now consolidate and work for improvement in whatever have been the gains in community care, which will be in users' interests, rather than move further down the road of privatisation as proposed by the Conservatives. But that is a general interest.

If such policies existed, what would they be? If we accept, as we must, that the mixed economy of welfare as created by the legislation is here to stay and that the state will not be clawing back powers of provision (as opposed to taking on a greater inspectorial, regulatory and monitoring role, as is likely), then what must be sought are those things which Conservative Government rhetoric promised but which practice has failed to deliver.

The need for a more diverse market of providers is not the main need. But even to achieve this is more difficult than it seems if we consider the lack of independent suppliers of services in some inner city areas (although this is where voluntary agencies are often strongly represented). But unless users have a real say in what services look like, it doesn't matter how many or how diverse they are. There should be a strong emphasis on advice, information and advocacy, assisted by implementation of sections 1–3 of the Disabled Persons (Representation) Act 1986. Another aspect of this would be the encouragement of more user-led organisations which provide services as part of that more varied market of providers. There is also a greater role for users in quality and inspection. The question here must be where these users are to come from. Too often the pool of people which a local authority draws on tends to be small and whatever efforts are made to enlarge it will come up against the fact that users have their own lives to live and they are not employed to be users (i.e. they are not 'professional' users). But in seeking to enlarge the pool of participating users and organisations, there is also a need to encourage organisers who represent, and are composed of, members of ethnic minority communities.

We have referred above to the problems of users playing the role designated for them in the drawing up of community care plans. In some ways this is one of the most urgent tasks and perhaps the easiest and least costly to bring about, as community care plans are the very foundation of the shape of community care in a local area.

There is also another kind of foundation and that is good social work practice. A great deal of user participation is about involvement in planning processes and research. For users to be involved in the machinery of decision-making would be a significant cultural shift. As Croft and Beresford (1996) state: 'Thus service users' main role in the development of modern  social work has remained essentially unchanged – to provide  information first for researchers and subsequently for social work agencies, policy makers and professionals.' But these writers also draw attention to the very basis of good practice – social work training and recruitment which socialise, as well as teach tomorrow's social worker. We know that this is important because of the research which has been carried out on what users expect from social workers. Beresford and Trevillion (1995) quote a service user with mental health problems who said: 'I think a lot of it is basic consideration for people. . . . It is treating people as individuals. Treat them as humans. It's all that sort of thing.' While Harding and Beresford (1996) refer to

> courtesy and respect, being treated as equals and as individuals, and as people who make their own decisions; they value people who are experienced and well informed, able to explain things clearly and without condescension and who 'really listen' and they value people who are able to act  effectively and make practical things happen.

Again, there should be no argument about this as it both stems from a basic humanistic approach and is also directly consistent with Biestek's principles. If users do not lay that foundation, then ideas of rights, participation and empowerment will remain no more than aspirations written on yellowing pages.

# Chapter 7

# Home from home?
## Residential care

**HOMES FOR CHILDREN AND ELDERLY PEOPLE**

Residential child care has its roots deep in the work of the Victorian philanthropists who founded Barnardo's, NCH Action For Children, the Children's Society and a host of other organisations, denominational and otherwise. Residential care for elderly people can be traced back to the Poor Law; indeed, it is not so many years ago many elderly people were cared for in what had been workhouses. Adams (1996) states that in 1960 37,000 elderly people were still living in former workhouses or other Poor Law accommodation.

There are other groups of people who live in residential care, mainly people with a learning difficulty and mentally ill people, but provision for them has sprung up in more recent years, occasioned by the closure of the old long-stay hospitals, the asylums of popular imagination. Certainly, the NHS and Community Care Act 1990 has caused a greater specialisation where the residential care of groups of service users, particularly that provided by private owners, is catered for.

But while residential care for elderly people and for children can be traced far into the past, in recent times their histories have been very different: most elderly people who today live in residential care do so in homes run privately, while there has been a dramatic shift in the way children are cared for. Only a minority now live in children's homes.

More than most other kinds of social care, residential care has tended to be viewed negatively by public and professionals alike. As Townsend has written:

> residential homes for the elderly serve functions for the wider

society and not only for their inmates. While accommodating only a tiny percentage of the elderly population, they symbolise the dependence of the elderly and their lack of access to equality of status.

(Townsend 1986)

Children's homes can also be said to confer the same low status, while their historical association with the orphanage nurtures the stigma of the abandoned and forgotten child whose sole source of care and shelter is the state or charity. Both children and elderly people living in residential care can appear to be rejected by the social unit which, culturally, is supposed to care for them: families.

Professionals are not immune to the prejudices of the general population but professional distaste for residential care can also be traced to the work of people like Ervin Goffman, who, in his book *Asylums* (Goffman 1962), constructed a critique of 'the total institution'. This had a profound effect on thinking about the long-stay hospitals and had much to do with the philosophical undermining of their *raison d'être*. And while the idea of the 'total institution' is applicable to a certain extent to those institutions, something of that criticism has rubbed off on professional attitudes towards residential care. Thus, for both the public and the professionals, residential care, for all kinds of groups, can look like a place of last resort.

The ambivalence which characterises our attitudes towards residential care (not somewhere where we want to end up but how is it to be avoided for others?) has left modern residential care tossed around on the tides of social policy. While there have been many advances in residential care in recent years it has yet to emerge from the long and seemingly unending period of neglect which gave rise to the government-sponsored Wagner review in 1986. The sector has been dogged for decades by widespread anxieties about its future, poor management, low morale, low-paid and (mainly) poorly and, in some cases, untrained staff. The Wagner Report (Wagner 1988), in the words of the title of its first volume, saw residential care as 'a positive choice'. But this is a cliché increasingly mouthed on conference platforms which often fails to be honoured in practice.

Changes in the numbers placed in children's homes and the proportion of qualified staff tell something of the story of that particular part of the residential sector. In 1992 there were about

15,000 places in children's homes, 10,000 of them in the public sector and the rest in the voluntary and private sectors. In the previous three years, the local authority sector had lost 2,500 places, the voluntary sector had lost some places and only the private sector was expanding (Warner 1992). A recent estimate puts the number of residential places in England at under 10,000, mainly in homes of 10–12 beds (Warner 1997). In 1992 there were about 15,000 staff working in English children's homes, a significant proportion of them agency staff. Some 13 per cent of heads of homes and 21 per cent of care staff in London boroughs came from agencies. About 80 per cent of care staff and about 40 per cent of heads of homes in local authority homes had no relevant qualification (Warner 1992). As Warner commented: 'Thus, there is no strong professional ethos around children's homes, as there would be with medicine or nursing, to act as a  partial safeguard against abuse and exploitation of vulnerable young people' (Warner 1997).

Even in the decade since Wagner reported, much has changed and, arguably, some of it for the worse. The general swing towards community-based services for both children and elderly people has increased uncertainties about the private sector's place and future.

Care for elderly people has been wrenched from its long mooring within local government into not-for-profit and private agencies. But the once-flourishing private residential sector has felt the cold blast of financial restriction as funds failed to flow so freely in its direction after the implementation of the NHS and Community Care Act in 1993.

Residential child care has decreased enormously in both the public and voluntary areas, with the rise of adoption and, particularly, with fostering and the consequent closure of homes. But it has also suffered from the unwelcome publicity that inevitably accompanies the gradual unfolding of scandals. The systematic and long-running regime of abuse by Frank Beck in Leicestershire and the so-called 'pin-down' regime in Staffordshire were the most publicised and sensational tips of icebergs that have come more and more into view. Widespread abuse, which may have involved hundreds of young people and dozens of staff as well as outsiders, in homes in north Wales was perhaps one of the most spectacular examples of what has come to light as the past has been ploughed up.

Not that these were the first scandals of modern times. In 1985 the Hughes Report on Kincora, a children's home in Northern Ireland, exposed widespread homosexual acts and prostitution in nine homes for boys in the Province. In South London, the Leeways Report showed a head of a home convicted in the mid-1980s of taking pornographic pictures of children in his care. And there were others. The public and the profession were shocked but it is only in the most recent years that there has grown a conviction that there may be something rotten in the state of residential child care that must be rooted out – that these abuses were not isolated or blemishes which the detection of perpetrators could remove. Better training, better management, changes to staff recruitment and selection, police checks – these are the barriers to stop those intent on abusing children and young people from infiltrating the homes, but only as effective as flimsy paper barricades against the onslaught of tanks.

Almost all of the incidents took place at least ten, or in some cases twenty or more years ago. But that is because it is almost inevitable that such scandals become public years after the events have occurred – vulnerable children in the 'care' of those who abuse them are not best placed to complain. As adults they may have the opportunity and the courage to do so. No-one would say that abuse does not occur in homes today. But the effect of these revelations has been to further demean residential care in the eyes not only of the public but of those who have responsibility for it – the immediate management of the local authority and, higher up, government.

Children are not, of course, the only victims of abuse in care. There is abuse of elderly people and of people with learning difficulties, occasionally even resulting in death. But this is much less well publicised than that of children and young people and also much less a matter of public concern, even if it has become more and more a subject of professional concern.

## GROWTH IN RESIDENTIAL CARE: PUBLIC TO PRIVATE

Yet residential care, despite the morass of problems in which it seems, for a quarter of a century or so, to have been entangled, did enjoy a brief but spectacular period of growth, or at least the sector for elderly people did. That growth came about in the early 1980s when the then Department of Health and Social Security amended the supplementary benefit regulations to make it easier for residents of private and voluntary sector homes on low incomes to claim their fees from the social security system. Assessment of financial need, not the need for such care, was what would determine public subsidy. As a result of this, costs to the public purse spiralled from £6 million in 1978 to £460 million in 1988 and £1.3 billion in 1991 (Walker 1992). The number of places in privately owned homes for older people and people with physical and mental disabilities (though the growth was largely for elderly people) almost doubled (increasing by 97 per cent) from 1979 to 1984 and by 1990 had risen by 130 per cent since 1979 (Walker 1992). Or, to use other figures, places rose from 46,900 in 1982 to 161,200 in 1991 (Laing and Buisson 1992).

There were influential effects of this. First, the very vulnerability of the client groups affected caused much attention to be focused on their care. The spectacular growth in numbers gave rise to concern about the quality of care and standards and fears that residents could be, or even were being, exploited for financial gain. The current emphasis on quality care, inspection and standards is directly attributable to that concern.

Second, the amount of public money haemorrhaging from its coffers alarmed the government. Six months after the Wagner Committee set to work in 1986, the Audit Commission published a report *Making a Reality of Community Care* (Audit Commission 1986), which drew sharp attention to the method of financing private residential care through the social security system.

The government acted immediately and appointed Sir Roy Griffiths to undertake a review of community care. Griffiths' critique (Griffiths 1988) not only focused on the obstacles to community care but showed a way out of the financial corner into which the government had painted itself. The government responded to Griffiths with a White Paper *Caring for People* (Department of Health 1989), which, in turn, led to the NHS and Community Care Act 1990. And while the Act's implementation was delayed for two years until 1993, the period between *Making a Reality of Community Care* and legislation passing onto the statute book, with the report and the White Paper wedged in between, was a remarkably short five years, given the scale of the changes which were ushered in – all of them with profound consequences for the size and governance of residential care.

Under the new legislation, local authorities would shift from being providers of care to purchasers of services from the independent (private and voluntary) sector. This, it was said, was a way of improving services, giving service users a choice, and tailoring services to meet the needs of those who used them. The way in which the new system would tailor services to people's needs was, in theory, that the users of services would go into residential care having been assessed as needing it. This was one of a range of possible options in an assessment process separate from actual entry into a home. For this to happen, social security funds were to be transferred to local authorities.

But there were serious consequences of the new financial arrangements for local authorities' own residential care (or, at least, that for elderly people). It was stipulated that 85 per cent of the funds to be transferred from social security had to be spent in the independent sector, partly due to the government's distaste for public provision and partly to stimulate a 'market' in social care. This meant that there was a financial imperative for local authorities to 'hive off' their residential provision into self-governing trusts, management buy-outs or the private sector.

The major transformation that was wrought can be seen in the fact that in 1976 for every one person accommodated in private care in England, five were in the public sector. By 1982 the ratio had moved from one to three, in 1988 it was one to one, and from 1989 the private sector came to dominate the market, so that in 1992 for every one public sector resident there were two in private care (Peace *et al.* 1997). On 31 March 1997, there were 307,000 places for adults in 23,100 residential care homes and 73,600 in 1,500 homes which were registered with both the local and health authority. The number of places increased by 11 per cent since 1994 to 513,200. The independent (private and voluntary) sector provided 88 per cent in 1994. Around 66 per cent of the 242,000 (149,000 in 1994) residents in residential care were in independent sector homes (41 per cent in 1994 and 20 per cent in 1993) (Department of Health 1997). Thus, in less than a decade, local authorities were transformed from being the major providers of residential home places to purchasers of them; and to inspectors, regulators and what the social work profession calls 'gatekeepers' – directing service users, through assessment and purchase, to different kinds of services.

However, there was an anomaly. Some local authority care was retained and private home owners complained (justly) that they had to pay fees to local authorities to inspect their homes, whereas homes run by that same local authority – alleged by the private sector often to be of a low standard – fell outside the scope of inspection. The eventual compromise (still a subject of debate) was the creation of so-called arm's-length inspectorates. When public homes were drawn within the inspectorial net (under the NHS and Community Care Act), the inspectors were part of social services departments, which were responsible for the management of local authority homes. Once the legislation applied equal standards in inspection, the pressure was on: expectations of higher standards increased and costs were squeezed.

The community care reforms have marked the biggest change to local authorities, in general, and residential care, in particular, in twenty-five years. But whether they have given the freedom of choice claimed for them, in this sector as in any other part of social care, remains an open question. The issue of charging for residential care is one which has come, since the reforms, to bedevil questions of choice. Charging residents for residential care has been the law since 1948. However, it is the very issue of choice which has brought the matter to a head. It has prompted the question of the extent to which those who are publicly subsidised when in residential care should be allowed to choose more expensive accommodation. The debate has centred on the principles exercised by local authorities to determine what is a reasonable cost. The government's guidance stated that 'the test should be whether the preferred accommodation is more expensive than the authority would usually expect to pay for someone with the same assessed needs as the individual concerned' (Department of Health 1992).

At the time of writing, there has been no resolution of this question. The Conservative Government, alerted to stories about elderly people's savings being whittled away in charges or homes sold to meet costs, rather than passed on to their children, introduced very complex rules about savings which, at the time of writing, local authorities are still challenging in the courts. The then Labour opposition promised a Royal Commission on long-term care, which was established when the party came to power. A large part of the commission's time will be taken up on this issue.

The community care changes and the arguments about charging have meant that many smaller private homes have become increasingly vulnerable as local authorities cannot afford to pay for care. This is not wholly a problem for the care of elderly people. Secure placements for young people in trouble can cost more than the fees at schools like Eton and Harrow.

More than many aspects of social care, residential care may often appear to present a depressing picture – some of its worst aspects seem resistant to change, the reality often does not match the fine words of reports and conference speakers and, in a social care field of general uncertainty, this seems to be the most uncertain part of all. But all is not lost. A great deal of private residential care is of a very high standard. The recognition that things must change is now accepted. While, for example, most of the recommendations of the Warner Report on staff recruitment and selection (Warner 1992), which came as a result of the Staffordshire 'pin-down' scandal, remain unimplemented, the strides made in inspection and quality assurance and standard setting could hardly have been predicted a decade ago.

The old virtual monopoly of the local authority has been broken but it has not been replaced by a private one, even though the private sector now dominates the elderly care market. Some local authority care for this group remains and there is some voluntary sector care. But a private market, unless dominated by a single supplier (as this market is not), is by its nature diverse. In 1980 Glomshire County Council offered forty homes but they were all local authority ones. Even if today Glomshire has none of its own to offer, five, ten, twenty or even forty different private owners may offer homes – and choice – in the county. And, in addition to that, there are now all kinds of community alternatives to residential care which eighteen years ago did not challenge local authority provision.

Choice may be more restricted than the authors and supporters of the community care reforms hoped but guidance, regulation and inspection, which must be seen in comparison with the comparatively minimal intervention and oversight which preceded them, have not only improved the quality of care but increased expectations.

Residential care has suffered greatly from the swing of the social policy pendulum. Its earliest status (in child care at least) was as a refuge run by people with a sense of vocation. In more recent times there came a recognition of its deficiencies which, in turn, led to something like a wholesale move against it, resulting in the large-scale closures of homes. This has meant that residential care of any kind now constitutes only a small part of the work of most local authority and voluntary sector child care services.

More recently there has come a glimmer of recognition that things have gone too far and that there will always be a need for a specialised service for some groups of people – whether they are deeply disturbed children who have never found a satisfactory foster placement and for whom adoptive homes cannot be found, a profoundly disabled person with learning difficulties, or an elderly person with severe dementia. But this kind of provision cannot be created on the cheap. It will need highly skilled, well-paid and extensively trained staff working in high-quality surroundings with high ratios of residents to staff.

The Wagner Report referred to the 'constantly shifting boundaries' of what constitutes residential care:

> with the emergence of new forms of provision: some of these, such as Very Sheltered Housing, Core and Cluster schemes, and multiple fostering are expressly designed with a view to combining the benefits of what have hitherto been considered separately as 'residential care' and 'care in the community'.
>
> (Wagner 1988)

These newer forms of residential care, if they can be called such, may well, in the not unforeseeable future, be the most common kinds of such care. Many would see them less as a fusion of 'residential care' and 'community care', as Wagner does, than as forms of community care. Questions of definition may not matter. How, for example, to describe group homes, which have replaced inferior care, like the long-stay hospitals, and, unlike their predecessors, are situated in ordinary streets, not hidden away behind walls and up long drives in rural areas? But in the foreseeable future it is residential care as is now most commonly recognised, residential care the heir of the 1970s' scandals and the 1990s' reforms, which will remain a subject of debate and controversy.

Residential care is not static – physically, in terms of the look and size of accommodation, it has been transformed. The population of those who live in residential care has changed: children are likely to be older and more likely to be damaged; elderly people are older, frailer and more likely to be confused. Regimes are different. The common currency of regimes today is about issues such as a concern for the rights of those who live in such care and the risks to which they can be exposed if they are to be enabled to lead as independent lives as possible.

And yet there is often something about residential care, at least for elderly people, which provokes resistance. As Peace *et al.* (1997) state:

> It can . . . be argued that the majority of older people, when they come to consider the options for coping as they become frailer in

old age, continue to put aside the residential option. Such sidelining is not because it is a glaringly cruel, institutional phenomenon; it is clearly not. We would argue that because residential care is still perceived as a serious threat to the self, potential residents are compelled to resist, even when the need for the benefits and supports on offer is  overwhelming. Losing individuality, even when losing control is accepted, is not to be countenanced.

The elderly persons' home, the children's home, as commonly understood – these and their descendants will continue be at the centre of debate. What place (if any) does such care have? What is to be the nature of their regimes? How are they to be financed? What rights are to be afforded to those who live in them? As residential care changes, even when it changes for the better, it continues to provoke such questions.

Chapter 8

# Something special
## Specialist services

**HOSPITAL SOCIAL WORK**

In the lady almoner and medical social work eras of social work in hospitals, hospitals were close-knit communities for both patients and staff. Length of stay did not seem to matter that much. Now each bed is a precious resource, needing to be freed for the next person to be bundled into it. In such a charged atmosphere, social workers in hospitals find themselves under tremendous pressure to speed up discharges by arranging instant community care services. Hospital discharge is the front-line of modern social services, with doctors and hospital managers often demanding the removal of patients into social services care. Social workers have to try to sort out the right arrangements for the patient, often having to brush aside unfair pressure if it will result in a doomed discharge and the likelihood of a swift readmission. Advocating for patients has to be balanced with the statutory responsibility placed on social workers under the 1977 National Health Service Act to co-operate with hospital staff. For the patients themselves, being back at home or away from a crowded hospital ward is invariably a better option.

Hospital social workers have to hop from ward to ward, assessing patients with an extraordinary range of needs. In seeking to arrange a safe return home for people with new disabilities, they have to make contact with a great number of agencies, many of whom themselves have no investment in responding quickly. Slowing down demand is in itself institutionalised. Co-ordination between hospital and community occupational therapists, or between hospital social workers and housing officers, is rarely as smooth as it should be. Above all, hospital social workers have to be great networkers. Some specialise on wards like rehabilitation wards.

Pre-natal hospital social work services are geared towards families where there is concern about the potential welfare of a new baby. Maternity social workers have little role to play in medical and technological decisions about embryo removal or selection of couples for fertility treatment, but they are involved once a parent and, indeed, all children in the family have been assessed as needing immediate support after giving birth. Concerns are mainly three-fold: if a mother is drug-dependent, the baby may start to experience withdrawal symptoms straight after birth; if there are child protection concerns, usually because of a history with a sibling; or if the child is not wanted, when the mother will receive counselling before and after birth about care options including family support, care by a relative in the short term, or adoption in occasional cases where a baby is totally rejected.

Boundary disputes characterise the management of hospital social workers. The local authority paying the salaries of hospital social workers will want to ensure that their own residents receive virtually all of that service, but in large teaching hospitals, in particular, many patients will come from outside the immediate area. As more hospitals close and those that remain serve populations larger than the average local authority, so hospital social work services will inevitably have to cater for patients beyond the local authority's boundary. GP fundholders also send patients outside their immediate area. Some groups of local authorities have established inter-borough agreements to reciprocate in the provision of hospital social work services. Some hospital social workers will carry out an initial assessment, asking the borough where the patient is usually resident to do everything else. Others, following a departmental instruction, refuse to see patients from other authorities unless it is an emergency. In some areas, hospital social workers have been pulled back to community bases, working in the hospital on a sessional and outreach basis.

## SOCIAL WORKERS IN PRIMARY CARE TEAMS

Many GPs would like their own social worker attached to their practice, as many of their patients have clear social as well as medical needs. In an ideal world, this makes sense. GPs are consulted by vulnerable people more than any other professional group, and are generally more trusted. GPs would like to have someone on hand who can help patients with the range of problems that social workers deal with. GPs and of course patients would get a faster more personal service that way. GPs and social workers working closely in tandem would be in a better position to detect and diagnose a number of complex problems and conditions that belie easy classification, such as the contributory causes of anxiety and depression, even of migraines, in the patient population. There is a case that more effective working together could contribute to reductions in prescribing, and more effective care. Practice-based social workers could also co-ordinate care to patients, making sure the principles of assessment and care management were more widely applied than they are at present. This would help to achieve more screening of over-75 year olds, one of the unmet objectives of community care legislation.

If it makes such sense, what's stopping it? Lack of resources is the main reason. There are not enough social workers to go round, and if social workers cover more than one practice, it is more sensible if they work from their own local base and share cover across the whole of the area with other social workers. That liaison-based approach can still enable GPs to make quicker and more effective referrals through their own liaison social worker, although shortages of resources will dictate that fewer referrals might be taken up. All referrals are usually offered an initial assessment under a liaison arrangement.

Another reason social services departments have not opted more for this arrangement is that budgets cannot easily be devolved down to social workers based in GP practices. Finance has to be held at an area-wide level, so that priorities can be worked out, especially as the managers with area-wide responsibility for budgets need the maximum flexibility in how they allocate resources.

## SOCIAL WORKERS IN HOSPICES

Approximately 270 hospice social workers across the UK belong to the Association of Hospice and Specialist Palliative Care Social Workers. British hospices provide terminal and palliative care to patients with cancer, degenerative diseases like motor neurone disease, and infectious diseases like AIDs. In the average twenty-bed hospice, three or four patients die weekly. Many patients are only there a matter of days before they die. Social workers have to be able to counsel patients and relatives within a period of hours or at most days, if that is all the time the patient has. Anxiety management, 'panic counselling' and bereavement counselling are the main skills required.

## SOCIAL WORKERS IN OTHER SETTINGS

Social workers are employed in a number of smaller settings, typically in ones and twos. These range from private sector commercial companies, where social workers carry out a staff welfare role; Ministry of Defence bases; specialist voluntary sector organisations such as Jewish Care and Norwood Child Care; and specialist directly run government services such as Glenthorne Youth Treatment Centre in Birmingham, and mother and baby units in women's prisons. Other specialist social workers include those who work with specific ethnic minority groups or with travelling communities. The professional training these social workers receive is exactly the same as that of mainstream social workers in the UK.

## SOCIAL WORKERS IN CHILD AND FAMILY CONSULTATION SERVICES

Social workers in the old child guidance clinics (now usually known as child and family consultation services) come from a long tradition of psychiatric social work, which used to have its own post-graduate qualification. Psychiatric social work used to be heavily psychodynamic, as that was the main theoretical background of other professional staff working in the clinics like child psychiatrists and child psychotherapists. The family therapy movement, including the various schools of therapy that arose in the 1970s and 1980s, was also highly influential. Recently, influences and methods have become more diverse, and staff in clinics have realised they need to work more closely with their funders, who tend to be a mixture of health, education and social services, and to respond with a greater sense of urgency to local social services teams, schools, residential homes, foster carers, and indeed to parents, so that their specialist help is given to children and young people in the community in greatest need. They used to be, and still are sometimes, criticised for choosing to work with the young people or families with whom there is the greatest chance of therapy succeeding. This does not go down too well with their funders, who want assessments undertaken, or therapeutic programmes established, for the most troubled young people and families they are dealing with, however grim the prospects.

Some regional or national specialist teams, such as the Great Ormond Street social work team, the Maudsley Hospital children's social work department, and the Tavistock Institute teams, are held in high esteem nationally and are consulted by social services departments up and down the country on particularly complex cases where local expertise is lacking.

## SOCIAL WORKERS IN BRITISH OVERSEAS TERRITORIES

Many British overseas territories have small social services departments. For example, the Cayman Islands has a department with thirty-five staff, and has a highly regarded low-cost family support service covering the island. Other former colonies such as Montserrat have regular contact with UK-based social services organisations, particularly for consultation. For example, one of the social services specialists at the auditors, KPMG, spent time in Montserrat advising the government there about how best to set up emergency shelters which were needed after repeated eruptions of the Soufriere Hills volcano. Similarly, social services staff have been called upon to advise in setting up new social services systems and new welfare agencies in a number of new countries without social institutions, such as Latvia and the Ukraine after the break-up of the USSR, and former military dictatorships where the role of the state needs to be consolidated to protect young democracies from further military take-overs or counter-revolutions. British social services is looked upon as a model of its kind.

## SOCIAL WORKERS IN SPECIAL HOSPITALS

From 1 April 1996, the three UK special hospitals, Rampton, Broadmoor and Ashworth, are now separate Special Hospital Authorities, each providing high-security psychiatric services to people who are especially dangerous or violent. They are provider services, whose services are purchased from the National High Security Psychiatric Services Board. About 70 per cent of patients at any one time are mentally disordered offenders referred through criminal courts or the prison service. The rest are referred directly from social services departments or health authorities, because of exceptionally challenging behaviours that cannot be contained in any other setting. A number of patients at special hospitals have a severe learning difficulty as well as mental health problems. All patients must fulfil the criteria in the Mental Health Act for compulsory admission.

The 1997 Crime Bill stipulates that once prisoners committed to hospital under hospital orders become well again, they must be transferred to prison to complete their sentence, rather than be rehabilitated into the community as at present. For staff as well as patients, this may well make rehabilitation-based social work a less attractive option.

## SOCIAL WORKERS' ROLE AFTER NATIONAL EMERGENCIES AND DISASTERS

Counselling disaster victims has become an important part of social workers' duties, and in every part of the country groups of social workers are on permanent stand-by. While they spend little, if any, time contemplating this, they do receive training in emergency planning, including graphic simulation exercises. When disaster strikes, counselling is a key emergency and follow-up service. 'The golden hour' after an emergency is when the main emergency services, the police, fire and ambulance services, have to co-ordinate action, save the lives that can be saved, and shift onto the site everyone who needs to be there. Immediately after many emergencies, there are distressed survivors. There are also relatives of people who have died tragically and unexpectedly. Both groups benefit from social work support, both in the aftermath of a disaster, and during the much longer period afterwards when grief continues rather than fades away quickly. After the fire in King's Cross Underground Station in London, a number of relatives were unnecessarily distressed by being given the wrong information about who had died and who had survived. Although Camden social workers were on the scene soon afterwards, it would have helped if they had been on the spot to assist with giving information and support to people as early as possible. After the *Marchioness* pleasure boat disaster in the River Thames, when over fifty partygoers were killed when the dredger *The Bowbelle* hit the boat, Southwark social services set up a helpline for friends and relatives. It was still going, and still receiving calls, for over two years before it was wound up. It was staffed by specially trained social workers on a rota basis. Social workers routinely attend distressing everyday disasters to provide counselling and practical support to traumatised victims or relatives and friends at the scene.

## EMERGENCY DUTY SOCIAL WORKERS

Between 9.00 a.m. and 5.00 p.m., five days a week, social services rely upon hundreds of staff to deliver a complex set of services. Between 5.00 or 6.00 in the evening and 9.00 the following morning, and all through the weekend, most departments have only a single duty officer available, from their emergency duty service. Most departments have a back-up pool, available at short notice, to come in and help if the shift is overwhelmed. People at risk in the night wait a very long time for a social worker to come. Social workers 'out of hours' deal with everything, and have to be particularly experienced in child care work and mental health work.

The job can be highly stressful, and officers are usually paid salary supplements to reflect the fact they have to make decisions without consultation or supervision, although *in extremis* they can contact senior officers by phone. Emergency duty social workers often receive so-called 'anxiety faxes' from day-time staff who are worried that a situation they have been involved in during the day might worsen in the evening or at night. Each emergency duty team (EDT) shift starts with a towering pile of such alerts.

Neighbouring authorities sometimes combine forces to provide a consortium emergency duty service. This can enable an EDT to be put together, which can give service users the choice of a male or female officer. This can be important in referrals like rape referrals. With a single-officer service, there is no choice. You get who you're given.

In future, it is likely the concept of a small out-of-hours service will give way to round-the-clock provision for specific care groups. Some community mental health teams already provide their own 24-hour cover. Adolescent care teams are moving in the same direction, as there is growing evidence that having a team of staff on stand-by to support young people at home can prevent admissions to residential care out of hours.

## INSPECTION AND REGISTRATION SERVICES

### Inspection services

Social services inspectors visit all residential homes in their area twice a year, once on an announced visit, and once unannounced. Their reports are public documents, and cover children's homes, residential homes for adults and 'dual registered' homes for adults which are residential homes with some nursing care beds. Nursing homes are registered and inspected by local health authorities, whose reports in general are shorter and will not be made public until April 1998. The current regulatory system is set out in the Children Act, law since 1991, the Community Homes Regulations (1991), also covering children, and the 1984 Registered Homes Act which regulates residential care for adults. Back-up guidance has been issued on the standards that should be expected, most noticeably in *Home Life: A Code of Practice for Residential Care*, published in 1984, updated by *A Better Home Life*, published in 1996, which was expanded to include nursing home care.[1, 2]

Since 1991, inspectors have worked in inspection units, which are meant to be at arm's-length from social services department operational management. However, teams of inspectors are still closely identified with the social services departments they work in. Home owners complain this is not fair and inspectors cannot be genuinely independent, as they would be if they were in a social services equivalent of Ofsted.

Social services inspectors also inspect some providers of children's day care, but while day nurseries, playgroups, crèches, after school playgroups and registered childminders are inspected as well as registered, other helpers such as au pairs and nannies are not regulated. In fact, nanny agencies were deregulated in 1995, although some voluntary registration schemes are available. There are 100,000 childminders in the UK providing 400,000 places, and about 17,000 playgroups also providing about 400,000 places. The standards of care are inevitably mixed. A small number of cases in which children have been killed by registered childminders have received national publicity, and these cases show up the limitations of the inspection and registration system. It can run basic checks such as police checks, and ensure an average standard is maintained, often through delivering training programmes. However, it cannot predict what will happen in the interaction between a child carer and a child during times of acute stress. That has to be a judgement exercised by parents. Some private detective agencies have sprung up as a result of recent publicity, offering services such as a week's covert surveillance of au pairs, nannies or child-minders, at a cost to the parent of around £600 per week. For this, the child carer is secretly filmed around the house so the parents can view the tapes and decide if they are satisfied with the standard of care.

Inspectors themselves need to have the mentality of detectives. While they are basically there to support and advise care providers, they must be aware that running care homes is a business like any other business. While the majority of care home owners behave with honesty and integrity, the market inevitably attracts the occasional pure profiteer and a range of holding companies owning more than one home who depend on the manager of the home to provide professional care and safeguards for vulnerable residents. If the manager is lax, or even worse an abuser, inspectors may be the only visitors trained to pick up warning signs that something is wrong. Their antennae have to be permanently attuned into the most awful possibilities. The power of home managers is considerable, especially in small private homes which are not part of any wider organisation. Staff and residents rarely feel they can challenge the authority of the manager, and in some cases, abusive cultures have continued for years, with powerful persuasive managers fooling inspectors. In some cases, managers like Tony Latham, who ushered in the coercive and brutal 'pin-down' methods in Staffordshire County Council children's homes, have been held up by senior managers and inspectors as professional paragons. A single inspector may be responsible for more than fifty homes. That size of workload means inspectors have to supplement their direct observations with the views of other professional staff in contact with local homes such as nursing staff, GPs and care managers, so that information about the standards operating can be collated and co-ordinated. Too often, the information held by care managers and social workers is held separately and not shared with inspectors, or notes are not compared across agencies.

Most homes for adults are in competition with one another for residents, whereas good children's homes are few and far between and can effectively name their price in a sellers' market. As in all businesses, market share is maintained by advertising, word-of-mouth recommendations and expediency – being in the right place at the right time when someone wants a service. Inspectors are supposed to be consulted by placement officers and care managers before a placement is made in a home in another part of the country, but this is not always done. Overall, inspectors have to win a battle of hearts and minds about standards. They have to be tough, as home owners can at times exert considerable pressure on them to write favourable reports. Inspectors have influenced care standards across the country for the better.

Lay assessor schemes are now quite widespread. This gives an opportunity to interested local people to join inspection teams after training. Lay assessors offer another perspective, especially if they have been service users themselves, or carers. The user community is still too rarely involved in setting standards for the services they use, which most other consumers of goods and services would be doing either directly or indirectly.

### Registration

Registration officers are inspectors with another hat on. They register all private care homes and private children's homes looking after more than four children. Local authority homes for adults and children do not have to be registered, although they are inspected under the common inspection regime. Registration officers have to go through copious checklists in which fifty or sixty questions are posed and answered, satisfying basic requirements like the physical condition of the home and the experience and qualifications of staff employed. This then counts as a benchmark against which future inspections can be measured. Inspectors try to gain a sense of what it is like to live in a particular home. A good question they can ask themselves is 'Would I like to live here myself?' or 'Would I like my mother to live here?' Inspectors also consider the effectiveness of the regime in a particular home. Does it promote as much independence as possible? Do individual residents have their own care plans or rehabilitation plans? Above all, is the quality of life of each individual resident in the home high? This is the vital question, as the worst homes in the country still run on 'warehousing' lines, with little concession to individual needs and lifestyles, and where activities for residents are organised on the basis of what is convenient for each shift. A star rating system similar to that used for hotels can help potential residents and their families to choose between care homes.

The 1996 Burgner Report, commissioned by the government, recommended substantial increases in the type of homes and services which should be subject to a formal registration requirement.[3] Burgner thought local authority homes for both children and adults should be registerable, so that there is a level playing field for all care homes and the private sector is not disadvantaged. If this proposal is implemented, substantial additional capital investment will be needed for all local authority homes across the country to be upgraded to registration standard, and this will inevitably lead to further closures and substantial transfers of homes to the private or voluntary sectors, because it is easier for them to raise capital. Burgner also recommended that small children's homes looking after fewer than four children, private home care agencies and private fostering agencies should all be subject to registration and national standards. Some services, such as day care for adults, and local authority in-house home care services, would still not be registerable. Partial coverage makes less sense than extending the regulatory regime to all who provide it, whatever the setting. This is likely to happen in due course.

The present system is widely felt to lack teeth, in that enforcement of standards and requirements can only be pursued through the courts with great difficulty. For those starting up a care home business, a local authority can rarely refuse a planning application and most test cases where a planning application has been contested have gone the way of the applicant. At the moment, providers play a cat and mouse game with inspectors. Private home owners challenge the rights of inspectors to insist on changes they have no wish to fund. Local authority providers challenge the view some inspectors take that some supported housing units are in fact really registered care homes because of the high levels of care being given. Overall, inspectors have influenced the overall standard of care for the better across the country just as much as a more heavy-handed legalistic regime would have done. It is their lack of perceived independence that recurs as a theme, although there is little hard evidence of them going soft on poor local authority homes. However, perceptions are important, and any potential conflict of interest would be removed by independence. The arguments against this are as compelling. A new organisation would need to be established with its own internal bureaucracy, which may not be financially justifiable without greater concerns in the future about the competency of inspection units than there are now. At present, there are probably enough checks and balances built in. Councillors see inspection reports at social services sub-committees. The reports are public documents. An advisory panel supports and monitors the local inspection and registration process.

There is a potential for duplication between local authority and health authority inspectors, especially as both register different aspects of the same dual registered residential and nursing home. Hertfordshire has a combined inspection unit which could become a trend.

# Chapter 9

# More than a piece of paper
## Social work training

## QUALIFICATIONS

It takes four years' training to become a senior librarian, nine years' to become a doctor, but only two years' to become a qualified social worker. The UK has a shorter training period for social workers than most other Western European countries. Despite considerable lobbying from within the profession and outside, culminating in a proposal for a three-year training period put forward in 1987, the government refused to extend the length of basic training up to that same three-year minimum prescribed by an EU directive for social workers across Europe.

The Diploma in Social Work (DipSW) is the professional qualification for all social workers in the UK and for probation officers in Northern Ireland (it ceased to be the recognised qualification for probation officers in England and Wales in 1995). DipSW, established in 1991, replaced the college-based Certificate of Qualification in Social Work, and the employment-based Certificate of Social Service, which were the standard qualifications in the 1970s and 1980s. Some professional staff now nearing retirement qualified with Home Office diplomas in the 1950s and 1960s and a few other historically obscure and superseded qualifications.

DipSW programmes, which attract student grants, are based at universities and colleges of higher education. There are over 100 programmes with an annual student intake of around 5,500, which is over 2,000 more than twenty years ago, although there are signs that the number of new entrants may be starting to decline. The options and combinations of subjects that can be studied at degree and post-graduate level have broadened out enormously in the last ten years. As with most other courses of study, students have the option of full-time or part-time study, or they can gain the social work qualification at home through a distance learning programme. While mature students can start the course without any academic qualifications, provided colleges are satisfied they can cope with the academic work involved, most students need either 2 A levels and 3 GCSEs in England and Wales, or 5 passes for the Scottish Certificate in Education, including 3 at Higher Level, or Level 3 GNVQ/GSVQ or NVQ/SVQ. It is preferable if applicants have already completed some relevant work experience or temporary work in a social work or social care setting. Many applicants are asked to go off and do this before applying when they make an initial inquiry. It is not yet clear whether the government's proposals to introduce and charge students for their tuition fees, and to reduce grants in favour of loans, will deter students in the future, especially as the long-term earnings potential of social workers is limited. They don't go into it for the money.

Social work training is regulated by the Central Council for Education and Training in Social Work (CCETSW). The chief executive of CCETSW reports both to the council itself and to the permanent secretary in the Department of Health. CCETSW is itself reviewed every five years, and is almost certain to become a national training organisation for the personal social services (TOPSS) by the year 2000, which will give it national workforce planning responsibilities.

The main thrust of the national training framework for social services staff, set out in 1991 in the *Personal Social Services Training Strategy*,[1] is to put in place a competency-based continuum of qualifications, going from fairly basic National Vocational Qualifications in social care for care staff, through specialist qualifications like the Certificate in Therapeutic Child Care, to the DipSW for social work staff and most managers, finishing with post-qualifying awards like the PQSW (Post Qualifying Award in Social Work) and the AASW (Advanced Award in Social Work) for experienced practitioners. The training continuum aims to give some training to all social services staff, over three-quarters of whom are unqualified, rather than just to put on better and better programmes for social workers and more senior staff. NVQs and post-qualifying awards are generally gained through work-based assessments, perhaps supplemented with day release at college. Employing agencies have to be fully committed to NVQ and post-qualification training, as considerable support for students is required, both in terms of identifying work-based placements, supervising students, and then assessing or 'validating' students if the agency has acquired assessment centre status.

More recently, employing agencies in conjunction with colleges are making the DipSW available to selected staff through an employment-based route, giving a combination of time off and sometimes small bursaries. Experienced staff may be able to complete the course quicker, by gaining credits under the Accreditation for Prior Learning system. This gives to mature and experienced staff who cannot afford to become full-time students a route by which to qualify.

The emphasis on competencies running through all contemporary training courses and programmes stemmed from a dissatisfaction by government and employers in the late 1980s and early 1990s that training providers were producing a generation of students who did not know enough about legal and professional issues when they finished their training. Professional training has to strike a delicate balance. Students must be taught about value systems such as anti-racism and anti-sexism, if their work is to be effective. They must also be helped to develop enough personal strength and confidence to withstand the pressures that will confront them once they start work. But like any pupils or students, they also have to be taught the basics, social work's 3 Rs. Margaret Yelloly believes NVQ training to be advantageous because 'it is relevant and meets the needs of the workplace, and has ethical advantages in making the criteria for assessment more transparent and open than has traditionally been the case'.[2]

All these qualifications (see Table 9.1) are competency-based, and the requisite core competencies are clearly set out for students and assessors in documents such as CCETSW's *Rules and Requirements for the Diploma in Social Work* (1991). Core competencies are quite general, like 'communicate and engage', 'promote and enable', 'assess and plan', 'intervene and provide services', and 'work in organisations'. The 1995 *Employment Survey of Newly Qualified Social Workers* found over 90 per cent of students were satisfied that the core competencies were closely matched with future job requirements.[3]

In general, students prefer placements to lectures and essays. Placements are where students cut their teeth, and gain a glimpse of what the job is about. CCETSW-approved practice teachers supervise students on placements, and they are usually experienced social

*Table 9.1* The continuum of qualifications

| Qualification | Definition |
| --- | --- |
| NVQ | National Vocational Qualifications, going from Level 1 to Level 5. Some trainees in supported employment go for Level 1, as might domestic staff like cooks. Levels 2 and 3 in social care are suitable for care staff in residential care and day care, and there is a Level 3 for advice work. Levels 4 and 5 are aimed at senior administrators and managers, and modules focus on business administration and all aspects of management. All NVQs are based on national occupational standards agreed by employer groups such as the Care Sector Consortium. |
| DipSW | The basic professional qualification in social work. |
| PQSW | The Post Qualifying Award in Social Work, commonly known as PQ, aimed at practitioners, recognising a higher level of skill and expertise. Most PQ awards are in child care, and in future a PQ award may become essential for staff working in certain areas like child protection work. |
| AASW | The Advanced Award in Social Work, recognising skills in policy making, leadership and management, but also in practice, i.e. the Advanced Award in Forensic Social Work. |

workers, residential workers or day care officers. There has been a continuous shortage of student placements for the last fifteen years, mainly because of pressure of work inside social work teams and agencies which limits their enthusiasm for taking on and supporting students. Students specialise in the second year of their DipSW, into an 'area of particular practice' such as children and families, elderly people, mental health, disability or learning difficulties. Other areas of particular practice, such as palliative care, are being developed by some colleges in partnership with specialist employers. Most students finish their DipSW course and gain the qualification without difficulty. Up to 90 per cent of newly qualified social workers find work within six months of qualifying. Invariably, a qualifying student's first job is in their chosen 'area of particular practice'.

Despite this healthy picture, Marsh and Triseliotis found that although there have been substantial improvements in social work education and training, there was a substantial gap between the needs of social work practice and the educational provision on courses. This study was also based on the views of newly qualified staff and supervisors! The concept of 'readiness to practice' was used, and whereas 80 per cent of new social workers felt ready, a comparable figure to other professions, only 50 per cent attributed this to any aspect of their course. The importance of a structured, supervised and well-supported first year of practice was emphasised in this study, as it seemed that a poor experience at college may be followed by poor induction, supervision and in-service training after starting work, at least for some students. This was especially true in social services departments, whereas qualifying probation officers fared much better back in the workplace.[4]

Specialist social services staff require other qualifications. In order to operate the formal sections of the Mental Health Act, social workers have to be approved social workers, and this involves successful completion of a 60-day specialist post-qualifying course with its own separate rules and requirements, based on 38 core competencies. Occupational therapists have their own professional Diploma. Accountants in social services usually have a professional qualification, and senior personnel staff would be expected to have the Institute of Personnel Diploma. Social services lawyers need to be qualified, and so on. As support staff in social services are devolved from central departments, so the onus is increasingly placed on social services to fund their training. Similarly, as the demands on support staff increase, it is essential for workforce planning purposes that they are accorded equal status with staff providing direct services to the public. This also means finding appropriate qualification pathways for computer specialists and administrators. The pace of change in the social services world is now so fast that new qualifications may be needed in new specialist areas such as commissioning and contracting, for staff to work effectively in these relatively new areas of responsibility. Jobs which are expanding way beyond their historical brief, such as inspection and registration work, would also benefit from a specialist training programme. Qualified staff also need top-up or refresher training. For many, their qualifying training took place in another era. Like bad drivers, some have acquired dreadful habits over the years.

## TRAINING

All social services departments have a training plan, which has to be submitted to the Department of Health who then allocate a Training Support Grant for social services staff to each local authority in the UK. Other agencies have to fund training out of their general grants and budgets. Training plans have to be developed after a training needs analysis, of individual staff, of staff groups, and of the needs of the service as a whole. Some training is mandatory, such as training in lifting and handling service users, which is part of a European Union health and safety directive. This is an expensive undertaking, as all home care workers and residential workers need to be trained.

Ideally, all organisations integrate training into a comprehensive human resources strategy. Each member of staff should have a training profile, as part of their own personal development plan. This in turn should be part of a performance management system, whereby targets are set and periodically measured for each member of staff. Targets should be based upon the organisation's priorities and action plans or business plan. Social services agencies tend to play this game at the organisational level and fail culpably at the individual level. Their plans, like community care plans and children's plans, make excellent, even if soporific, reading. However, apart from a handful of dedicated supervisors, few agencies put the same level of effort into planning for individual members of staff, unless they are staff with problems who tend to receive a disproportionate amount of attention in order to dot the i's and cross the t's before shifting them out of the workforce.

An analysis of who gets training in social work agencies tends to show that while some staff put themselves forward for lots, others get none at all. Sometimes, provider-led courses are put on with no reference to a training needs analysis simply because an in-house trainer has an expertise in a particular area. Often, the staff who need training most avoid it at all costs as part of their general strategy to evade scrutiny. If there is a problem, or a crisis, in an agency, a training programme is rapidly devised and money thrown at it as part of 'action-plan-itis'. It is no surprise that the underlying endemic problems that caused the crisis remain obdurately resistant to change. Training may be part of a solution to problems, but changes in management are just as important and usually have to be made first.

Some social services agencies now adopt a broader approach to training and development, both in content and method. For instance, *A Change of Mind*, written by Peter Spafford, is a searing 1-hour play about the impact of Alzheimer's disease on a family. A theatre company performed it to staff groups around the UK in 1997, and then took it on an international tour. As a training event, the play showed to up to 300 staff at a time in different organisations for under £1,000 a show, and in one hour conveyed all you need to know about Alzheimer's. It was an exciting and cost-effective form of training that also brought staff together across agencies. Too many training programmes are confined to one agency. Services often fail because the boundaries between agencies are not broken down. Training is a good way of stretching boundaries. While they should not fund all of it, social services should take a responsibility for making sure training takes place locally across sectors, and that staff from different agencies, including the independent sector, are able to participate in programmes. This is part of a responsibility for standards across sectors.

Innovative thinking about training is greatly needed if outcomes are to be improved. One-third of social workers' time is spent in cars, so the Personal Social Services Research Unit at Kent University is designing research audiotapes for social workers to listen to while they are driving around. Research is given insufficient weight in training programmes. Training programmes have a tendency to put the form before the content. Learning to communicate better is one thing, but what you communicate is more important. Hard presentations of research are rarely given, and these would be better than the lukewarm snippets of low-level information often given out by 'touchy feely' trainers who prefer to think their own insights hold the ultimate value, or worse that the participants' off-the-cuff insights are worth more than they really are.

The social care organisation of the future will be a learning one. It will rely upon its own staff rather than external consultants. It will seek to rebuild the camaraderie lost during the cold excesses of some public sector business planning regimes. Openness, respect and trust will become the buzz words. The job needs to be both interesting and enjoyable, and the key to this is staff development. There are ways in which the continuum of qualifications can benefit both in-house students and their teachers. NVQs in business administration raise the skills not just of the administrative staff working towards the qualification, but the skills of other staff involved either as assessors or internal verifiers, if the agency is accredited as an assessment centre. When a change programme is established, small focused project teams can be set up using internal staff with an emphasis on staff development as well as task completion. Internal secondment programmes can give staff experience of working in completely different jobs in the same department. This can broaden understanding and break down barriers, as when a fieldwork manager is seconded to run a residential home and vice versa. Struggling individual staff can be offered specialist one-to-one coaching for a period of time, as part of their own training needs development plan. The coach can be another member of staff for whom that too will be valuable additional experience. A dynamic training and development programme, when mapped out, should include at least a quarter of the total number of staff in the organisation, and this should be rotated every two years so that over an 8–10-year period all long-term members of staff gain from the programme. Such a programme also increases the promotion prospects of ambitious staff. A broad approach to training is more than a piece of paper to say you have qualified.

Service users can also make use of good training programmes, where the support and advice of specialist training staff is vital. Foster carers can undertake NVQ training, and people with learning difficulties can go on courses as diverse as an NVQ in fast food delivery.

# Chapter 10

# The manager's tale
## Management of social services

The general shift in UK companies and organisations during the 1980s and the 1990s towards a culture of management, and a focus on raising the quality of public services, has made life easier for today's social services managers. The power bases of the main public sector union Unison were systematically neutralised during the Thatcherite era of union-bashing, although the public sector resisted this onslaught the longest. By the early 1990s, managers were back in the driving seat, a position some had not properly occupied since the early 1980s. The balance has now tipped the other way. Standing up for staff in the late 1990s can in some authorities attract the same looks of contempt as being a manager used to do a decade ago, when management was a dirty word. Elsewhere, a more caring model of management is striving to withstand the onslaught of crude business ethics, an obsession with performance management as the cure for all evils, and trendy designer models of management imported without being customised for local use from America and Japan. The same debate about how to raise standards within education goes on within social services. 'Making progress through praise' has its supporters, but so does use of a competency-based approach to sack underperforming staff. A 1997 European Commission Green Paper 'Partnership for a new organisation of work'[1] emphasises the need for modern organisations to be based on 'high skill, high trust and high quality'. Social services is unsure about the kind of organisation it should become.

Welfare agencies reflect business trends. Staff reduction means there are fewer managers in most departments, and those remaining have larger teams and wider responsibility. Removing tiers of management and devolution mean greater powers and decision-making have been delegated. Support services have usually been the first casualties in cuts rounds, so as to leave the maximum number of staff on the front line to carry out direct work. It looks as if political short-sightedness has gone too far and led to a stripping out of infrastructures, depriving those managers who are left of the very tools they need to manage rapid organisational change. Unlike their continental counterparts, few social services managers keep within the maximum 48-hour working week defined in the European Working Time Directive. Most work beyond the scope set out in their job description.

About 10–12 per cent of all social services staff hold a management position, although junior managers often work directly with service users in addition to supervising staff. Unlike the health service, social services has no regional or national management structure, in which managers with potential are identified early, fast-tracked through management development programmes, and regularly promoted, within a national policy framework. There is a strong social services community, but one that carries more a sense of cumulative history than a clear vision of the future.

Social services management still sits uneasily within the overall management of local government, as ambivalent about being inside the structure of local councils as education managers are. While some years ago there was a fear within the profession that general managers from companies like BP or Sainsbury's would be shipped in to shake things up, very few such appointments have been made. Most shortlists for senior management posts are still made up of qualified social workers who have risen through the ranks. The interview format has changed, however. Whereas ten years ago a new director of social services could be appointed after an hour-long interview, today's senior appointments tend to be made at assessment centres lasting two or three days, with many of the candidates on final shortlists having been discretely head-hunted.

Local authorities, particularly new chief executives, typically want to reorganise councils from within while social services legislation pushes departments outwards towards health agencies and the voluntary sector. In fact, strategic alliances between departments within councils are just as important to good social services as thriving external partnerships. This tension between whether to realign social services departments within the council or with external agencies, particularly health agencies, needs to be understood and cleverly managed. It is no surprise that managers experience change fatigue with pulls in so many directions. A number of management consultants are now advising authorities that changing   structures will only have a marginal influence on service improvement and the organisation's culture and style. They emphasise that managers have to be subtle and sophisticated, rather than macho and buccaneer. Companies such as Levi Strauss say it takes 10–15 years to achieve a real turnaround in an organisation, way beyond the time public sector managers are usually given. This time scale is judged to be realistic by Daphne Statham, Director of the National Institute of Social Work, writing in 1996, when she suggested that

> bedding down the current changes within the social services field will probably take another decade, leaving aside the impact created by changes taking place in the context in which social services operate, and, more broadly, at the European and international levels.[2]

However, in local government, four years, the life of a local political administration, is usually regarded as more than enough time to do everything. Indeed, most restructurings are undertaken primarily to get rid of managers currently in post, with short-term agendas to the forefront. Restructuring remains the most legally fireproof way of clearing out management teams and creating a different climate. Margaret Thatcher is quoted by Francis Pym as regularly asking Conservative MPs 'Are you one of us?'. Attempting to create a united management team of like-minded people is another loosely trumpeted goal of reorganisations, but change alone may not be worth the months or years of planning blight and low morale it brings in its wake. The danger in perpetual upheaval and change is that a group of middle and senior managers cut themselves off from work and staff on the ground. By doing so they can create a self-fulfilling parallel organisation, a virtual social services department, which is then unable to impact much on the very front-line standards it came into being to overhaul.

Feeling at home in your immediate work team, enjoying contact with service users, and feeling supported by your immediate manager, are the three biggest factors in staff morale. Working in a good team with a good manager means that whatever is happening in the rest of the organisation doesn't matter quite as much. The best managers and management teams create an aura around the workplace and their organisation, command respect from all quarters and attract great loyalty from their staff, who in turn work their socks off. Support for first-line managers is essential, as they are sandwiched between pressure from above to achieve change, and pressure from below in relation to managing the demands of a front-line service.

In Chapter 3, we described how the relationships between local councillors and social services senior managers are critical to how well social services departments function. The best councils maintain stability even during intense political change. Other councils are known either for their blame cultures, for their ideological obsessions, or for an ultimately destructive political instability. During a long period spanning the 1970s, 1980s and 1990s, the London Borough of Hackney, in north east London, combined all three features. The following case study illustrates the impact of local politics on a department and its services. The impact of key individuals is a rarely appreciated but significant factor.

## CASE STUDY: HACKNEY SOCIAL SERVICES

It is hard to evaluate social services departments before the mid-1980s when external inspections began in earnest. Nowadays it's hard to move without bumping into auditors or inspectors, some of whom seem to be in virtually permanent residence. Hackney had a reasonable reputation, and in the early 1980s its director of social services, Mary Sugden, was elected by fellow directors as President of the Association of Directors of Social Services. In 1982, she crowned a distinguished career by moving on to be the principal of the National Institute for Social Work before retiring.

Some local Labour Party activists were happy to see her go. Many of those activists were also staff in Hackney social services. Others were local councillors. This was the age before the Widdicombe proposals were introduced in 1988, which prevented senior local government managers also standing and serving as councillors, a move felt by some to lead swiftly to a devastating reduction in the ability level of the average local politician, and by others to herald a relative de-politicisation of local councils. Many activists in the Hackney Labour Party in the early 1980s were local government officers in other councils. Hackney is one of the poorest and most socially deprived areas in the UK, and is ethnically diverse with over 100 languages spoken. Black children in care formed a disproportionately high group within the overall numbers of children in care, and most black children were left for years in mediocre or dreadful out-of-borough residential placements and foster homes. Those who wanted to see Sugden go felt her regime of professional social work served Hackney's needs poorly. They may have been right, but as Dr Johnson said, 'the road to hell is paved with good intentions'.[3]

They looked around and in 1983 selected Gordon Peters as their new Director of social services. Peters, a left-wing academic, whose only jobs in social services up until then had been as an unqualified social worker and research officer in a neighbouring borough, Islington, was immediately faced with a number of strikes as NALGO flexed its muscle to see if he was really on their side, even camping out in his office for days during one dispute so he had to work from an alternative location. NALGO usually had the support of the majority of local councillors, so although he was left wing, Peters found himself faced down by *ad hoc* alliances of union activists and councillors.

It was not surprising that the managers underneath him felt unsupported, and a number of professional staff left in despair or were pushed out as the department became more politicised. Some groups of staff continue to meet ten to fifteen years later, initially in support groups fused together in anger, later in friendship groups who still retain an interest in what was happening in the department which had been such a powerful working experience for them, both good and bad. In the mid-1980s, the Chair of social services at the time, Patrick Kodikara, became very involved in the direct running of the department, and appointed a number of staff who, like Peters, held no professional qualification. Kodikara felt that to hold a professional qualification was a form of contamination and signified an inability to understand the needs of local black people. He thought Hackney Council, as well as social work courses, were racist, and that this situation could only be changed through a takeover of recruitment practices. The up-side of this policy was that in an area with high levels of unemployment, the council, as the biggest local employer, acted responsibly to create as many jobs for local people as possible. There is an echo of this approach in the 1997 Labour Government's welfare to work programme. However, in Hackney social services, whatever its theoretical underpinning, the policy went wrong. Critics claimed that to live locally and to be black became as important a factor in recruitment decisions as being able to demonstrate professional skills or attributes. Whatever its racial motivation, the strategy led to large numbers of unqualified local people being appointed, who were immediately offered long-term employment protection because of the council's no compulsory redundancy policy. The least capable members of staff of all races who were fundamentally incapable were sent on a merry-go-round of redeployments, weakening each service they worked in. Managers of services had no say in the staff they were given, as personnel staff had been given complete responsibility for the redeployment process. Peters was very much part of this era, and indeed regarded a low pay deal he introduced as one of his greatest achievements. In later years this deal became something of an albatross, as it was the main reason why Hackney's home care service became prohibitively expensive. In many ways the undoubted advances made in the 1980s, such as the better deal for black children in care, on its own a massive achievement, were undermined by a lack of attention to basic systems and practices.

Gordon Peters resigned as Director of Hackney social services in 1990, possibly sensing the unease in the Labour Party under its new leader John McCafferty about past excesses. McCafferty appointed a new director, Joyce Moseley. Moseley was a career social services manager whose brief was to turn what had become a catastrophic situation around. At the time she started, in February 1991, the departmental budget was overspending by several million pounds, and the legacy of politicisation remained, in that several staff were suspended, some for over two years without their cases coming to a disciplinary hearing. Morale was rock bottom. During the preceding period, of course, it had not been all bad. Pockets of good practice existed, but general professional standards had deteriorated to the point where, in 1989, the Social Services Inspectorate felt it necessary to monitor regularly the general performance of the department. These misgivings were echoed eight years later by the incoming Labour Government which openly and publicly threatened to send in the hit squads to recalcitrant social services departments who received dire inspection reports from the Joint Review Team (see Chapter 3).

Between 1991 and 1994 Hackney social services concentrated more on improving services than being perpetually diverted into politics. Such was the degree of service improvement that some services were externally recognised as state-of-the-art for the time, although to some extent managers had begun to champion innovative projects at the expense of investing in mainstream services. In 1994, Hackney fostered the second highest percentage of children in its care of all UK councils. Only Gwynedd in North Wales, with a much smaller group of children, fostered a higher percentage. Four years before, Hackney's performance had been one of the worst in the country. The process of service development was helped by the chief executive at the time, Jerry White, who later went on to become the Ombudsman for Southern England. White introduced a service planning process council-wide, backed up by centralised procedures. He pursued his vision with the same ideological zeal about his product as Kodikara had done before him on the member side. However, White rejected attempts to modernise personnel procedures into a human resources framework with an emphasis on devolution, performance management and performance appraisal. Shortly before leaving, he realised that the model of which he was so proud was being overtaken by a new wave of managerialism based on devolution and empowerment, changes which new community care legislation typified. In the early to mid-1990s under Moseley and the Chair of social services Sharon Patrick, the political and professional arms of the council worked well together, much as they did in the Kodikara/Peters era. A number of black staff were dismissed, and this led to renewed allegations by local activists and staff within the council that what was being done was racist, especially the reversal of some of the policies of the late 1980s. Moseley and her managers were emotively accused by the trade unions of 'ethnic cleansing', a term used to describe genocide in Bosnia in the conflict between the Serbs and Croats in the early to mid-1990s. Hackney had a higher proportion of industrial tribunal cases on the go than any other council. By 1994, Hackney social services had been a political and personnel battleground for a decade.

But just as the department, especially those staff who were having to cope with the pressures of new legislation and considerable increases in the volume of work, longed for a period of calm, a new political storm gathered. In a coup within the Labour group, Sharon Patrick was replaced as Chair of social services by a new member of the Labour Group, Hettie Peters, who had been a councillor for less than 18 months. She was the first black Chair since Patrick Kodikara. Sharon Patrick was marginalised and Peters quickly took a dislike of Moseley, perhaps for being the archetypal professional, white, middle-class woman. The parallel with Mary Sugden twelve years before was uncanny. Like Sugden, Moseley was elected as President of the Association of Directors of Social Services, but before she could take up her position in October 1997, she was made redundant. The two years between 1995 and 1997 were as politically charged as anything in the 1980s, and illustrated the potential for political intrigue and agendas to destabilise public services like social services over and over again. So, what happened in the two years between Hettie Peters being elected Chair and Moseley being made redundant?

Peters was being formally advised by Demetrious Panton, who Hackney Council had appointed as a policy adviser. Panton had been in care to Islington council and had received £15,000 in an out-of-court settlement after suing them for being sexually abused in a local children's home. Multiple abuse in Islington children's homes had been the subject of separate independent inquiries by Emlyn Cassam, the former Director of Norfolk social services, and Ian White, the Director of Hertfordshire social services. The London *Evening Standard* had done much to expose the abuse scandals, and to support Panton. Panton advised Peters how best to conduct a campaign she was keen on furthering in London local government circles, warning against the evils of paedophiles. In November 1995, Peters herself was charged with housing benefit fraud. The charges against her were eventually dropped, and she made counter-allegations of conspiracy against her political opponents.

At about the same time, a former Hackney social worker who had died of AIDS, Mark Trotter, was at the centre of allegations that he had abused children in Hackney's care, who themselves could have become infected with the virus as a result. 'Trottergate', as it became known, was the trigger for one of the worst political splits in the history of Labour groups. Seventeen Labour councillors, including Hettie Peters, formed a breakaway group and started to vote with the local Conservatives and Liberal Democrats. Officials from the national Labour Party tried to build bridges, but to no avail. The Labour administration collapsed and the seventeen rebel councillors were formally expelled from the national Party, whose rules state they could not reapply for membership for at least five years.

By this time, Jerry White had left as Chief Executive to be replaced by Tony Elliston. An ambitious general manager, Elliston began to rubbish all that had gone before him and slated Hackney's services for being some of the worst in the country. Like many directors in post, Moseley found it difficult to embrace his agenda of 'transforming Hackney' with the total ideological commitment he demanded, taking the view that not all of Hackney's services were bad, that some were considerably better than they used to be, and that he was promoting a negative blame culture. Elliston thought that attitude amounted to lame incrementalism, and recommended a new management structure for Hackney to councillors, which abolished all director posts, including Moseley's post as Director of social services. The structure was approved by the new administration, using the votes of the Labour rebels. Moseley took early retirement. Under Elliston's new plan, all Hackney social services senior managers were made redundant, and new ones appointed. Elliston himself was accused of getting rid of staff, including many black staff, an echo of past accusations against others. The industrial tribunal cases kept coming, including one brought by the former Head of the Press Office, Mick Gosling, who had once been a high-profile trade union convenor at Fords in Dagenham, and another by the only black director of education in the country, Gus John. Elliston claimed nothing short of the action he proposed would guarantee local tax-payers improved services. A possible fresh but more secret ideological agenda was to contract out many services to the private sector. While he quickly became a guru to a small band of enthusiasts, the general morale of the organisation, and certainly that of social services, plummeted. New managers coming in said they were determined to sort it all out, just as other new managers had pledged years before. Managers who were once seen as part of the solution were now defined as part of the problem. The majority of staff felt that popular competent managers had been replaced for political and ideological reasons, in acts of betrayal and revenge the outside world, in the shape of the Department of Health, knew about, but made little effort to stop. This was possibly because the independent inquiry into the handling of the Trotter affair, conducted by the ex-Cambridgeshire chief executive, John Barratt, was under way at the time. No-one in government wanted to take a risk by supporting in public managers they were commending in private. Just before the 1998 council elections, most of the seventeen Labour rebels cynically switched to other political parties such as the Liberal Democrats and Conservatives in order to maximise their chances of being re-elected. The Barratt report concluded that while some individual managers made mistakes in their handling of the Trotter case, the political climate was too Machiavellian for a professional culture to survive within it.[4]

Hackney has never been an easy place in which to work. Over the years some of the best brains in the British public service have worked there, cutting their teeth before moving on to better jobs and higher salaries. Some brilliant teachers worked at Hackney Downs School over the years, and the closure of the school in 1995 in a blaze of publicity and recriminations after even a government task force found it could not turn it around, does not invalidate the contribution made by many people to maintaining or raising standards. Their contribution is often ignored or dismissed.

The saga of Hackney social services is not unique. Similar machinations can be found in many councils across the UK, although they represent the worst excesses rather than the general state of play. They form a powerful argument that far from local government being a positive democratic process, it can hamper the efficient management and delivery of services. While government by quango or regional administration may not be the solution, because of the removal of key public services from the control of locally elected councillors, some safeguards against undue political interference in the professional delivery of services are advisable. Concerns should not be confined to Labour local authorities. A friend of one of the authors, when working as a senior manager in a flagship Conservative authority, had it suggested to him that it would be made worth his while if he were to write a report, over the head of his director, recommending to councillors that the authority's residential provision be transferred to private sector care organisations.

All management decisions are made within a political framework. In a health authority known to one of the authors, the decision about where to site a new hospital was effectively taken at the local masonic lodge to which a majority of leading board members and clinicians belonged. The decision to save St Thomas's Hospital rather than Guy's in the London Hospitals Review conducted by Sir Bernard Tomlinson in the early 1990s was a political one. St Thomas's connects by an underground tunnel to the Houses of Parliament. The chief executive of the health authority responsible was visited by the head of the Secret Intelligence Service, as well as other politicians, and was told which way the decision needed to go – for security reasons.

The point about political interference is that it is only one of a number of factors which can destabilise the energy and creativity of managers and management teams. The challenges facing today's social services managers are immense, and there is a sense in which management always feels like a race against time. In large public sector bureaucracies, getting things done is by no means easy, and considerable management skill is needed to solve everyday problems or confront vested interests, many of which have resisted change for years. The list of achievements of social services managers is an impressive one in the last ten years, including implementing major budget reductions, implementing major new legislation like the Children Act and the NHS and Community Care Act, including taking on major new responsibilities, and supporting the growth of the independent sector which has now if anything become over-stretched.

## DAY IN THE LIFE OF A SOCIAL SERVICES MANAGER

The following diary extract is an account by one of the authors of the issues facing a social services manager, designed to draw out the excitement, the drama and the sheer variety involved in managing social services.

It is a wet November Sunday morning. My phone rings. A manager of a day centre for people with learning difficulties tells me some gypsies have parked their caravans on the centre's forecourt, blocking the entrance. She has explained to them the purpose of the centre, but that has not deterred them and more caravans are arriving by the minute. I advise her we can ask the police to move them on, but that we better wait until tomorrow to check the council legally owns the forecourt. We decide to close the centre tomorrow as a precautionary measure, so that the coaches ferrying users in to the centre don't get blocked in and so the users aren't subject to any stress if the police are involved and things get ugly. Three hours later, the manager rings me back to say she's persuaded the convoy to move on by herself. I forget to ask her what she's doing there on a Sunday. The answer would be taking responsibility. Many of our staff continue to be involved with service users out of hours, on an unpaid basis, such is their commitment.

This incident also illustrates the strength of a social services structure. We have always placed an emphasis on supervision and teamwork, unlike some professions like district nursing where there is a flaky structure of supervision and management. For example, district nurses are frequently left to their own devices with only their professional training to fall back on. In the social services community, there is always someone to ring and consult.

Later on that Sunday, I go through my in-tray. There is good news about the coming winter. The government has just announced an extra allocation of money for social services to relieve pressures on hospital beds. We will spend it on extra staff for our home from hospital team, so that when elderly people leave hospital there is a check made that they can cope, that relatives and neighbours are informed, and so that there is someone to come in and make a cup of tea. Putting the bid for the funding together involved meeting with health authority senior staff at short notice to review the overall resource position, including backlogs, waiting lists and pressure points. We get on well, and quickly identify areas of common concern. The Secretary of State talks of a 'Berlin Wall' between health and social services but our partnership is an honest and productive one, without any turf wars.

We are reviewing every service in the department, and that level of change is difficult for staff. Dealing more effectively with the present brings uncertainty about the future. We have a number of problems to tackle, including assessing people for simple requests much quicker than we do at present; reducing some wild variations in service levels such as long waiting lists in one part of the borough and none in another part; and connecting up the experiences of users with our strategies. Internally, if the planning for new services is done properly, the new arrangements will readily be agreed by staff, politicians and trade unions. The key is consultation. If as managers we consult properly, and if we are prepared to amend grossly unpopular proposals, we can make the sorts of changes to services by consent that would have been unimaginable ten years ago.

I look at a new set of performance indicators. They show that in the last year we advised or provided services for over 18,000 people, about 1 in 8 of the local population. That advice or direct provision will primarily have been given out by our 200 front-line staff, which means each of them will on average have supported about 900 people in varying degrees of need or distress. Of those 18,000 users, 120 complained, less than 1 in 150. Those figures represent a substantial contribution to community organisation and relief of poverty and misery. Nationally, since the start of the community care reforms in 1993, social services departments have carried out over 100,000 community care assessments and 20,000 assessments of the needs of carers. The workload has been massive. Between 1993 and 1995, there were 620,000 new referrals for occupational therapy. I try to think of ways we can publicise this invisibly accumulated track record. The only times the local press have shown interest is when our staff pulled out all the stops during a civil emergency, when an unexploded World War 2 bomb was dug up, or when something has gone wrong, big-time, in a child care or mental health case. We have had about five such cases in the last year, which I would say is a good record of achievement rather than a stick to beat us with.

Valuing staff is a big issue. However much we try, staff complain we're developing a workaholic culture that's a bit macho, in which it's getting harder to admit mistakes. This is the very opposite of what we intended, and it must mean we have to work harder or smarter at communicating with staff, even about why certain staff get suspended or sacked from time to time. When this happens, the fear and blame side of things can get out of hand. We need to explain that raising standards involves tough action, but that doesn't mean any less support for staff.

I look at the diary for the coming week. Tomorrow I'm touring our sheltered housing blocks with the Director of Housing, to see if we can develop some of the most run-down units into a positive and less expensive option than additional residential homes. Later in the week, I'll be chairing a meeting with education staff to carry forward our plan to set up an early intervention scheme in primary and junior schools, where we are trying to intensively support troubled children before it is too late. I'll also be seeing a number of external auditors who are coming to inspect some of our services as part of their routine programme. I'm also half-way through an annual visiting programme to all our staff groups and local voluntary organisations. This week there are four such visits, which I do to stay in touch. There'll be the odd crisis this week, as there is every week, but nothing we won't be able to deal with. The aspect of it I worry about most is that with so much going on, it's easy for someone like me to take my eye off the ball, to not attribute sufficient weight and time to perhaps a small issue which if it is not dealt with quickly, can get out of hand. But I have a good management team around me, and between us all, we usually manage to cover everything. The job's exciting and interesting, a real privilege to be doing.

## WOMEN IN MANAGEMENT

Despite women managers at the highest level having a long and honourable history in social services, management remains firmly a male prerogative. Not only are women managers a statistical minority – over 80 per cent of directors of social services are male, an inverse proportion to the percentage of men working in the most junior positions – but male managers still hog the stage. This can be literal, as when male managers seek to dominate conferences and other public forums, clamouring for airtime, irrespective of whether they have anything to say. All managers need to be tough, but women managers need to be hard as nails to handle sexism in its contemporary elusive manifestations. A number of women in management programmes have been developed by universities, and networks of women managers are in place in some parts of the country. Women have suffered in the general move away from equal opportunities issues in the 1990s. The creation of new unitary authorities in Wales in the mid-1990s resulted in only one woman director of social services out of twenty-two being appointed, a worsening percentage.

## BLACK MANAGERS

What is true for women managers is magnified for black managers in social services. Look around any room of managers and there'll be one-third less black faces than five years ago. While there are reasons for every separate resignation, appointment, retirement and promotion to managerial ranks, the overall situation can only be explained by institutional racism. Even if large numbers of black managers decided social services wasn't for them, or if large numbers were displaced having been over-promoted in the first place, little has been done either to recruit new black managers in the same numbers, or to maintain a commitment to existing black managers and to train them and support them to do the job better. In some urban authorities, this 'whitening' of the management structure, which John Le Carré calls 'altitude sickness',[5] has been almost violent in the speed with which it has happened. This may also reflect black networks offering mutual advice about where to work and where not to work, and where the 'glass ceilings' are worst. Many black managers who have left social services have found other high-level work such as lecturing or running black businesses. It is not as if they were incompetent and have ended up as gardeners or shop assistants. It will be harder than ever second time round to build groups of black managers back up to a level in the workforce which is proportionate to local population patterns. It could only be done with systematic management development programmes for junior black staff, which will be expensive and unlikely to find political favour in these harder performance-obsessed times. Junior black staff may themselves be ambivalent. Seeing all-white teams above them, and seeing what happened to their colleagues who made the same journey a decade ago, they may say no. In August 1997, an industrial tribunal in North London found Brent social services guilty of racial discrimination against seven staff, most of whom were 'unfairly selected for redundancy', in a flawed selection process used to 'remove black staff who were considered to be difficult'.

# Chapter 11

# Acts of charity
## The role of the voluntary sector

## CHANGES IN THE VOLUNTARY SECTOR

In less than a decade the voluntary or charitable sector threw off the last vestiges of philanthropy and the do-gooder and was transformed into a major industry. As a whole (that is the totality of the voluntary sector, not just that offering social and welfare services), the sector now accounts for just under 2 per cent of Gross Domestic Product, receives total voluntary income of £268 million a year, employs equivalent to 440,000 full-time staff and supports approximately 2 million volunteers. While the sector has seen an increase in central government funding, the financial contribution made by local government has steadily increased. In 1992 the sector received £588 million from local government and this had increased by 15 per cent by 1995 to £687 million (Hanvey and Philpot 1996b).

However, the sector remains extraordinarily diverse, something which the figures quoted above tend to disguise. For example, the majority of charities are small, with 88 per cent having income of no more than £100,000. Conversely, a small percentage of charities control the majority of the sector's gross income.

What the sector does is also varied. There are local voluntary bodies, largely composed of volunteers. A parish church, used only by worshippers twenty years ago, might well now offer a base to a mental health drop-in project and an AIDS support group. There are other local groups, often staffed by volunteers, with loose attachments to well-resourced national bodies like Age Concern and Mind. Then there are the large national charities providing highly professional services, staffed by paid workers (but also using volunteers) and supplying services for groups as diverse as elderly people with dementia, children in trouble with the law and people with a severe learning difficulty. These groups may (like national Mind and Age Concern) or may not have a lobbying, campaigning and advocacy role.

These varied roles account, in part, for the different degrees of dependence on grants, fees and charges from charity to charity. Mind's proportion of income from these sources is 29 per cent, while Community Integrated Care, which was set up to provide services under contract, receives 99.4 per cent. Scope's income from fees and charges grew from 53.7 per cent in 1991 to 64.1 per cent in 1994, while Sense's went from 51.4 per cent to 68.9 per cent over the same period (*Henderson's Top 2000 Charities* 1995).

The welfare arm of the voluntary sector has, perhaps, changed more than the rest. As far as child care is concerned, all child care charities but, most notably, the big three – Barnardo's, NCH Action For Children and The Children's Society – underwent a massive shift in the kind of care provided. All had begun by mainly (but not only) providing care in homes (see Chapter 1). By 1990 that had become a very small part of their provision and, where it existed, tended to be very specialised and very different from the large and institutional orphanages with which they had traditionally been associated. For example, NCH Action For Children (then the National Children's Home) had thirty-nine residential homes and eight residential schools in 1974 but only four family centres and three hostels for young people leaving care. Twenty years later it has 215 projects but residential homes and schools, now offering highly specialised care, now numbered only twelve. Among the rest were 23 independence projects for young people leaving care and young homeless people, 23 community-based young offender and youth projects, 15 counselling, advice and mediation projects and four homefinding services. Treatment centres for children who had been sexually abused had grown to 14, while there were 21 services for disabled children (Philpot 1994a).

But the most far-reaching promoter of change for all social services voluntary organisations – from those working with children to those working with elderly people, from learning difficulties to physical disability – has been the community care reforms, proposed by the Griffiths Report (1988). The government's social security policies had created a mushrooming private residential sector that grew, in cost to the Exchequer, from £6 million in 1978 to £1.3 billion in 1991 (Walker 1992). The quantitative effects of this can be seen in the fact that between 1981 and 1991 the number of elderly people in local authority homes fell by 20 per cent and the numbers in homes run by the private and voluntary sector rose by 300 per cent (Adams 1996).

It was this unpredicted and unbridled growth in the costs of private residential care that formed the original impetus to the appointment by the government of Sir Roy Griffiths to undertake his review. He was asked 'to review the way in which public funds are used to support community care policy and to advise . . . on the options for action that would improve the use of these funds as a contribution to a more effective community care'.

Hard on the heels of the Griffiths Report came the government's response a year later, the White Paper *Caring for People* (Department of Health 1989), which was then given legislative sanction by the National Health Service and Community Care Act 1990, implemented in 1993. The White Paper, among other things, proposed the idea of care packages (a range of services designed to meet the needs of individuals to allow them to live as independently as possible in their own homes) based on the professional assessment of the needs of individuals, while services would be based on those needs (needs-led services) rather than on what was available to provide them (resource-led services). Such an approach, said the White Paper, would 'make use wherever possible of services from the voluntary, "not-for-profit" and private providers insofar as this represents cost-effective care choice'. Social services departments were to become 'enablers' (and purchasers) rather than direct providers of services. They were, therefore, expected 'to take all reasonable steps to secure diversity of provision' and 'in particular, they should consider how they will encourage diversification in the non-residential care sector'.

Thus, the concept of the mixed economy of care was born. This now common term 'is used to distinguish the complex pattern of statutory, voluntary, private and informal provision from the simple pattern of state and local authority services which was a widespread principle after the welfare state of 1945' (Adams 1996).

## MIXED ECONOMY OF CARE

However, despite claims that social services departments were monopoly providers of care, the reality was otherwise and there had always been a mixed economy – meals-on-wheels services had been largely purchased from bodies like Age Concern and the Women's

Royal Voluntary Service and local authorities had often bought places in homes run by the large voluntary organisations. In most towns and villages, but especially in urban areas, hundreds of small voluntary organisations and groups keep going on a shoestring, funded by donations and small grants given by individuals, companies and institutions like banks and councils. Between them, they provide a broad spectrum of social care services at a negligible cost. And 'informal' care which family members and others provide for disabled relatives must not be overlooked.

What the National Health Service and Community Care Act did, apart from giving a stimulus to expand the role of the voluntary sector in welfare provision (and, by so doing, diminish that of local authorities), was to consolidate a much more formal relationship and partnership between the sectors.

But while the new system grew in part from a deep-seated dislike on the part of a right-wing government of publicly provided services and local government, and its need to cut public spending, it is also true that the philosophy behind what were to become the reforms had found favour on the left. Indeed, as long ago as 1985 (that is three years before Griffiths reported and five years before the legislation passed on to the statute book), George and Wilding, two writers associated with the academic left, wrote:

> For the New Right, the mixed economy of welfare is a euphemism for cuts in public provision. For the socialist, the term describes a new pattern of partnership between statutory and voluntary, formal and informal, family and state welfare. . . . A genuine partnership between statutory and non-statutory and family norms of social care is the most effective method of providing adequate services.
>
> (George and Wilding 1985)

What has been described as 'a major cultural shift for both local authorities and voluntary sector organisations' (Means and Smith 1994) was outlined in detail in the White Paper, and in the legislation and the guidance which accompanied it (see Chapters 5 and 6). To promote the new mixed economy and the welfare market, the government designed financial arrangements in such a way that local authorities were encouraged to buy services from the voluntary and private sectors, rather than provide them themselves. The Act made it compulsory for every local authority to spend 85 per cent of the Special Transitional Grant (that is, the social security monies spent by the government on private residential care placements which would move to local authorities to spend on the new system) on the 'independent sector' – services provided by private and voluntary sector agencies (see Chapters 5, 6 and 7). It was financially disadvantageous for a local authority to refer people to its own homes. Thus, many authorities were encouraged to 'hive off' some of their services – particularly homes for elderly people. They were turned into non-profit-making trusts so that they could compete with providers in the voluntary and private sectors. One effect of this attempt to create competitiveness with the voluntary and private sector was that the so-called market in social care services was stimulated. However, for most users of services, choice is illusory in that either sufficient variety does not exist within their area from which to choose, and/or local authorities, as the purchasers of services, cannot afford the fees demanded by suppliers.

There remain other problems with this market. One of these is that it is notoriously unstable and insecure with providers. Both the private and voluntary sector, who 'diversified' (that is, started providing services which had not been traditionally theirs), find themselves moving in and out of financial crisis and dependent on the whims of purchasers – who are *not* service users.

Another problem with the market is its unevenness. For example, while in inner city areas one is hard put to find private residential homes for elderly people, this kind of provision is highly concentrated in seaside resorts. The private sector in domiciliary care is less well developed, with a few large suppliers and many small ones. This was something which the White Paper recognised when it stated, wishing to encourage local authorities to create diversification in the non-residential sector, that one of its key objectives was 'to promote the development of a flourishing independent sector alongside good quality public services'.

All this, of course, begs the question of whether voluntary organisations *should* succumb to the blandishments and financial temptations proffered by government to become major providers of those services which have traditionally been largely the preserve of local authorities. But voluntary agencies are also mirroring local authority provision in the field of services for children and families, where the 85 per cent rule does not apply, purely because of financial pressure on those authorities. If the dividing line between statutory and voluntary sector becomes blurred – and no government can now turn back the tide of the mixed economy, even though it might be frozen – who will fund and promote the innovative services which had often been the prerogative of the voluntary sector before such services became part of the mainstream of provision?

With the state stimulating the sector and the demands placed upon it by entering into contracts to provide services, will there be a Darwinian fight for survival with the weakest (that is, less financially stable) charities going to the wall? Will access to services diminish and greater choice prove an illusion as larger providers, less interested in innovation and more attuned to the need to maximise income, push smaller ones to the margins and even out of business? This tension is already evident when a large national provider of nursing home care moves into an area and undercuts the prices of small local homes.

The Deakin Commission (National Commission on the Future of the Voluntary Sector 1996) proposed a 'concordat' between the voluntary sector and central government to recognise and ensure the sector's independence. However, two problems arise from this. First, it is local government contracts (albeit at the behest of central government) which potentially threaten independence. Second, it is arguable that the voluntary sector is too diverse and fragmented to be drawn into an over-arching, binding agreement, even one which appears to be in its favour. Indeed, it was the argument about diversity which persuaded the then Heritage Secretary Virginia Bottomley to dismiss the idea of the concordat.

If the state is to cede large parts of its responsibilities to the sector, this raises questions about how accountable services can be, and the changing and deepening responsibilities of trustees. Just like elected members of local authorities, trustees are faced with complex decisions and issues that intimately affect vulnerable people and their communities. Trustees may find themselves responsible for multi-million pound structures with additional and complex investment portfolios. But while the local authority member is accountable at the ballot box and, in many large local authorities, may be more or less part-time (albeit supported by expenses), few, if any, trustees are anything like full-time and – importantly – the boards on which they sit are answerable to no one but themselves. As Hanvey and Philpot have written: 'Replacing themselves in their own image, often not reflecting our society's cultural diversity, sometimes unsure of the boundaries between policy and management issues and free to follow whimsical inclinations, trustees sometimes present a worrying picture of the sector' (1996b).

The questions of how voluntary agencies can become meaning-fully accountable or how boards of trustees can be democratised are rarely addressed. Instead, the questions arising from the sector's new role tend to be answered only partially in terms of the control and monitoring of services. Indeed, in introducing the legislation, the government emphasised that one of the new roles for local authorities was not just that of enabler but also co-ordinator and regulator of services. A welfare state is one where the state takes central responsibility for ensuring the security and well-being of its citizens without discrimination, on the basis of civil rights and with the optimum consistency of standards across the country. The state is concerned with equity and entitlement, but we know that even nationally provided services cannot guarantee this. The National Health Service is based upon the principle of being free at the point of access on the basis of need. Yet variations exist throughout the country in terms of, for example, lengths of waiting lists or the length of stay in hospital for maternity confinements.

The quality of services, and how those services are provided, have become increasingly a matter of government and public concern the more the market has diversified. The role of the local authority as planner, co-ordinator, purchaser and monitor of services has become more and more important.

The example of the USA can offer some insight here. Not because it can be defined as a welfare state but because its social care provision is so much more diverse, its systems so much more complex and its standards so often more wanting than in the UK. Harding and Phillips have written of the problems of a market system for the long-term care for elderly people:

> Where the market exists, however, the worst effects have been mitigated by a firm system of local planning, based on a shared value base, which has controlled, regulated and developed local services. The [few] areas where such local planning exists can demonstrate greater consumer satisfaction, greater equity of access and better cost control and value for money.
>
> (Harding and Phillips 1996)

The USA has a longer history of the contract culture than the UK. Gutch (1992) found that voluntary organisations became less, rather than more, financially secure as a result of short-term renewable contracts. He also remarked on the generation of paperwork and bureaucracy; the greater power of professionals and full-time workers against that of volunteers; an increase in commercialism and competitive behaviour among voluntary agencies; and that competition had been used to reduce costs and contracting had concentrated on the purchase of provision rather than on whether the service user benefited. His other findings were that he could draw no strong conclusion that organisations became distorted as a result of contracting; but that small organisations were tending to be squeezed out as the larger ones could better afford to 'play the contracting game'.

Studies in the UK confirm such fears for this country and also draw attention to fears about the impact of contracting on innovation, the growth of dependence, and the impact on the structures of voluntary agencies (Flynn 1996). Indeed, there are examples of some of these fears being realised. Flynn (1996) gives an example of how one drug and alcohol charity, motivated by the offer of contracts, moved into the field of caring for people with long-term mental health problems.

James Richardson's survey (Richardson 1995) found that only 11 per cent of contracts were written by purchasers, while 15 per cent of those he looked at were written by the provider and the rest produced jointly. He noted some change in the nature of services but that these were caused by need and demand, not by the imposition of contracts. He commented:

> None of the results [of the survey] provided support for the hypothesis that contracting has led to significant interference in the nature of service provision through the medium of contracting ... the survey suggests that fears of widespread mission distortion have not been fulfilled.
>
> (Richardson 1995)

Again, fears about the effects on innovation were not borne out. Osborne (1994) found that voluntary agencies which were mainly funded by the public sector were not less likely to be innovative. Only 39 per cent of the organisations who relied on voluntary contributions in this study had developed innovations; the 74 per cent of those who relied on public funds had developed innovations.

Flynn (1996) believes, following other studies, that the distortion which will occur in the sector overall is the squeezing out of smaller bodies serving less popular causes, rather than distortions within individual bodies. He says that this is because transaction costs for the purchaser are higher, the smaller the contracts which have to be negotiated and monitored. They take up more time and resources to negotiate. Larger contracts are cheaper to negotiate and it is less risky to manage service delivery through contracts with large and established agencies. But this in itself could negatively affect innovation in that smaller bodies often have come into being specifically to innovate in areas of specialised need. Also, while bodies like Barnardo's and NCH Action For Children are centrally directed, the branches of Age Concern and Mind are not – they are, in effect, as far as negotiations are concerned, autonomous local bodies.

When it comes to financial stability, Flynn also found that increased income from contracts was not as healthy as it may seem at first sight. This was because competitive tendering can lead to unrealistic bidding with no certainty that the winners will be able to deliver within the price bid. This can lead to attempts to renegotiate contracts or cut costs so that quality suffers. Flynn adds that assumptions are made by bidding providers about the numbers of future users with whom they will work. If these are not maintained financial instability can result. He quotes Richardson (1995) as finding that services have had to be changed, not because of purchasers' preferences, but through changes in demand.

There are also other financial considerations which can impact negatively on voluntary agencies in the contracting process. Not least is the effect of the instability for staff in particular and future direction in general under a regime based on short fixed-term contracts. These create uncertainty and make it difficult to develop and retain staff.

Opportunism can be another consequence of contracting. An organisation can build up a collection of contracts over a relatively short period. These may, positively, generate income. Negatively, they may move the direction of the body away from its original intentions but without much concept of where it is going. Russell *et al.* discuss this from their survey:

> None of the sample appear to have defined a strategic view of their future role to [*sic*] this changing environment. The question of whether the organisation has a development plan elicited a negative response in all but one case. Given the voluntary sector's history of having to work from year to year, this is perhaps hardly surprising.
>
> (Russell *et al.* 1995)

Of course, a variety of contracts may both give financial stability and prevent dependence on any one purchaser but to seek to develop in this way demands strategic thinking rather than taking chances as and when they come. A balance must be struck between flexibility which purchasers seek and the stability required by providers. Flynn and Hurley (1993) believed this contradiction to be inherent and Flynn (1996) has said that the problem remains and that stability for providers can only be achieved with long-term contracts.

But whatever the positive or disadvantageous effects of contracting, what they cannot do is redress the inequalities within the welfare system, or iron out the imbalance of power and information between contracting parties. The smaller the voluntary agency is, then the greater that imbalance. However, flexibility is also desirable within voluntary organisations. Contracting could well impose a uniform approach by the voluntary agency, leaving its regions and branches without freedom of action to negotiate on their own behalf.

Another development of recent years has been the growth of self-help groups, not simply groups of service users promoting their own cause but ones actually providing services to meet the needs of their members. On the one hand, such developments provide a welcome invigoration of the sector, offering new initiatives and a break from traditional roles. But, on the other hand, as Mayo states:

> Neither equal opportunities specifically, nor community partici-
> pation, community development and self-help more generally,
> can simply be left to the operations of the free market . . . there is
> no reason to suppose that, left to themselves, such organisations
> will be able to continue to operate at their present level, let alone
> play a more significant role in the direct provision of services. On
> the contrary, there is evidence from the experiences of organisa-
> tions in the USA to suggest that contracting services out to the
> voluntary sector, in the current context of the mixed economy of
> welfare, may strengthen the largest and the best established
> organisations but at the potential cost of pressurising them into
> adopting increasingly commercial and/or bureaucratised ways of
> operating. Meanwhile the smaller, more directly community-
> based organisations may be far less able to participate in the
> mixed economy of welfare.
>
> (Mayo 1994)

So far the questions raised have been about the effect on service provision of creating a mixed economy of welfare. At the end of the day is the service user better off? Can the level of services be maintained? As the public sector recedes, will the voluntary sector take on care for, and work with, the groups which attract less funding and public sympathy?

The relationship between the voluntary and statutory sectors since the legislation has taken effect has proven less fraught than was at first feared. But this does not mean dangers are not still present and may not yet arise. However, we are talking about a massive change in thinking and operating. There are people not yet in positions of influence who are growing up with the new culture and will become leaders of both sectors in the future. Their experience, their lack of attachment to old (but not necessarily worse) ways and values may yet have an impact. In the meantime enough has been discovered about what some of the effects are or might be to give reason for caution. A continuing period of financial stringency for the statutory sector, with its impact on the voluntary sector, may mean less of a wish for give and take, less of an ability to see the position of the other side, and more of a tendency to grab what one can when one can.

## THE FUTURE OF THE VOLUNTARY SECTOR

There are two other large question marks which hang over the sector – the effect of the National Lottery and the fall in voluntary donations. The National Council for Voluntary Organisations has claimed that the Lottery is responsible for a 11 per cent fall in individual giving (and a net loss of more than £300 million in individual donations)[1] (Etherington 1996). It may, in fact, be too soon to tell what the long-term effect on individual giving will be, even if one accepts these interim figures.

But even before the Lottery, charities were feeling the cold, with the failure of planned, tax-efficient giving to increase proportionally in this decade. It remains at about 10 per cent of total giving and seems unlikely to increase without government encouragement through more tax concessions and better promotion. Etherington (1996) believes that it is difficult to see any increase in the numbers of people giving by tax-efficient means in the foreseeable future, and points out that, in fact, donations have fallen from £1.40 a month in 1987 to £1.28 a month in 1993. 'Increasing economic insecurity,

limited growth rates and a propensity to spend on other activity'
indicate, he suggests, that matters will not change for the better.
While paying tribute to the Charities Aid Foundation for encouraging government to provide increased tax concessions, Etherington
states:

> While this work has been important, the general lack of recogni-
> tion by the public of a civil responsibility to give may ultimately
> have resulted in very limited change. The public has very clear
> views about what charities should provide. British Social
> Attitude Surveys have continually revealed that charities have a
> distinctive role that is not connected to basic provision. This may
> ultimately be a major constraint on the public's propensity to
> give.

(Etherington 1996)

Etherington does not go on to the logical conclusion that if this is
so, the situation can only worsen if voluntary agencies, through the
new community care system, take on more of the responsibilities
which have traditionally fallen to local authorities, of which some
are basic provision.

It is beyond doubt that the National Lottery Charities Board,
together with the four other lottery boards and the Wellcome Trust,
will determine much of the future shape of the sector. Yet there is
virtually no public debate about whether short-term funding for
designated programmes, designed to meet the needs of, among
others, poor people and children, is a healthy way for the sector to
develop.

The new community care system has largely replaced grant aid
for the sector with contracts by local authorities. Contracts tie the
sector to work in certain ways with certain groups. Arguably, they
diminish both independence and innovation. The other large source
of charitable income is from individuals, through legacies, fund
raising and planned giving. It is arguable that this source is a guar-
antor of independence and gives freedom to innovate. Yet, the
NCVO's doom-laden statistic about individual giving aside, it is
predicted that legacy income will fall (for NCH Action For
Children alone that represents £4 million of its £14.5 million annual
voluntary income (Philpot 1994a). Even before the Lottery was
launched, planned tax-efficient giving had not increased propor-
tionately over the past five years. These facts alone offer a challenge
to the health and future of the sector.

The community care reforms have created new structures within social services and social work departments built on purchaser and provider functions, the creation of care managers, and the development of assessment skills. But many problems have arisen to frustrate the intentions of the reforms. Perhaps the greatest of these, which goes to the very heart of the reforms, is that the hoped-for assessments based on the needs of the users of services have been turned into budget-driven ones. This has meant that the criteria on which services are made available have been drawn tighter and tighter and, as a result, more and more people have been denied services of which they are in need, a situation which has been often challenged in the courts.

According to the rationale of the reforms, critical to needs-led assessments is the opportunity for choice for the users of services and choice is itself posited on the idea of a market in social care. This market remains unevenly spread geographically.

The new arrangements had gone too far to be disentangled (even if that were desirable) by the Labour Government. What their effects will be on the welfare of the individuals they were introduced to serve is unclear and will remain so for some while. As Chou En-lai said, when asked to assess the effects of the French Revolution: 'It is too early to tell.'

# Chapter 12

# All in it together
## Working with different agencies

The general public and politicians rightly expect social care agencies to work well together, and are understandably exasperated when they don't. The Labour Government came into power determined to reduce youth crime, and indeed many individual local authorities had been giving a high priority to collaboration and partnership working in this area for some years already. However, evaluations of joint working arrangements in youth justice carried out by the Audit Commission in 1997 suggested that despite the efforts and entreaties, little had changed, and the requisite co-operation, both at a strategic and operational level, remained patchy.[1] It looks as if the current government, like previous governments, will have to be prepared for a long haul if one of its central objectives of improved joint working is to be realised. The inter-agency world in social care is notorious for the gap between its strategies, of which there are many, and their implementation, where only a few agencies have comprehensively broken with tradition.

In August 1997, a 5-year-old boy, Dillon Hull, was shot through the head at close range by a gunman in Bolton. He had been out with his father, a local drug dealer, who was probably the intended victim in a drug war contract hit. Dillon's mother was addicted to heroin. Her younger child Codie was born addicted. Neither child was on the local child protection register, but social services both in Blackburn and Bolton were aware of the family and their drug misuse. After Dillon's death, the age-old question was asked: should he have been removed from his parents? It goes without saying that had he been he would still be alive. Yet both his mother and her partner loved Dillon and looked after him well enough in the circumstances. The case is a reminder of the dilemmas social services and other agencies face every day, in terms of what they tell each other, and what action they take.

If agencies do develop integrated working patterns, they increase the chance that in the most alarming situations, which are a minority, they will be able to act together effectively. Good communication lies at the heart of successful inter-agency working. For example, different professionals visiting someone vulnerable can record the time of their visits, and exactly what they did, in a notebook that is always left in the flat or house as a permanent case record. This can act as a medium both to exchange information, and to co-ordinate help and avoid duplication. Each professional can also alert others to a particular need or worry. This is a simple way to assist effective joint working, worked out and carried through by staff on the ground.

For social workers and other public sector professionals working in social care, it is always hard to know what is going on. The police clear up less than 1 in 5 known serious crimes at best, and a much smaller percentage of overall crime, which includes estimates of undetected crime. They increasingly rely upon paid informants for the information to make arrests and secure convictions. Social services has no tradition of paid informants. Generally speaking, the people they need to acquire information about are people shunned by their communities. If a man who is either drunk or going mad stands in your street in the middle of the night screaming, or charges repeatedly at your front door in the mistaken belief he or a close buddy lives there, you will call the police, pray they come quickly to take him away, and not worry too much about what they do with him. If you see the man again, you will probably turn your head away, even if you furtively glance back. It's unlikely you'll make a point of seeing if he's OK and alerting your local social services department if you're worried. Similarly, the man himself is unlikely to ask for help when he needs it most.

There is a view expressed by some that in the circumstances outlined, agencies have to be seen to take some action, even if they know it will be ineffective, because less blame is attached to action than inaction. At worst then, we have a professional environment in which the crucial information is often missing, and in which the wrong action may be taken either as a result of poor information, or defensively in order to be seen to be doing something. There is a clear danger that professionals might act in a populist way when feeling under threat themselves. Strong management support is needed if staff are to feel confident enough to take professionally sound but personally brave decisions.

So what about paid informants, paid according to the quality of their product? This would go against all principles of normalisation and encouraging positive attitudes towards marginalised people. It would encourage snooping, snitching and suspecting the worst, especially if there is a reward attached. A balanced approach is better. The Benefits Agency has a freephone to report suspected fraud, where information can be left anonymously. Social services departments can set up public helplines with a freephone on which concerns about all vulnerable people can be phoned in. A permanent message can be printed in local newspapers, worded like:

> If you are worried about a child at risk, or elderly person in trouble on their own, or if someone who seems to be mentally ill may need support, phone social services in confidence on ... Your information can be handled confidentially, and anonymously if preferred.

The action taken on the information provided should always be proportionate. Senior managers and politicians have to be prepared to carry on explaining to a sceptical audience over and over again why decisions have and haven't been taken, and to anticipate the demands from the public and press to be open and honest. A sense of perspective has to be kept. Most decisions made are sound and would attract public support. Although results of user satisfaction surveys use different methodologies and sometimes produce conflicting results, the majority of surveys reveal a high degree of satisfaction by a consistent 80 per cent of users of social services, one of the highest satisfaction levels for a public service.

Generally speaking, agencies providing social services are working better together. The average social services department has an average of over sixty planning-level relationships with other agencies for children's services alone.[2] Whereas a few years ago, you could put representatives of different organisations in the same room, and they'd argue, disagree and jostle for position, nowadays it's more likely the same group will look for a common purpose in dealing with a mutual problem. There has been discussion of introducing a formal qualification in multi-agency work. There is also a growing realisation that blaming exercises are short-sighted and a sign of organisational immaturity. When social workers think of blaming the police for not responding quickly enough in the middle of the night to a call, it helps if the police explain to them how few patrol cars they have operating at 4 in the morning these days covering huge geographical areas in crime terms.

Integrated services are springing up everywhere, although it may take some of them years to be more than a group of strangers from different agencies sitting next to each other at new desks with nothing much else changed. Many joint initiatives are inevitably savings-driven, and this can sometimes obscure the core separate function each agency is responsible for, which can get lost in the excitement, anticipation and potential of merging. Better co-ordination or outright integration are not made any easier by frequency of staff changes. Joint teams often have a 50 per cent turnover every two to three years. Working relationships between agencies have to be re-established over and over again. It is likely more examples of collaboration or outright merger across agencies will take place in the next 5–10 years, in the quest to reduce management costs, and to provide more co-ordinated services.

Working together doesn't come naturally or easily. Each separate agency has an overwhelming internal agenda which can be more pressing. For instance, by 1997, health authorities were required to let the Secretary of State know their 600 priorities. Each agency faces a complex annual budget-making process, staff shortages at the operational level, day-to-day crises, and a permanent reorganising climate. Surviving 'change fatigue' and meeting internal priorities can be an achievement in itself and can exhaust the last ounce of personal and organisational energy. Serious collaboration with a partner agency can still seem a desirable but not an essential objective. The service might be simple but the working relationships are complex, especially where there is more than one professional culture involved. Faced with internal pressures, or just through habit or laziness, one agency can ignore its partner agencies altogether.

Pooling budgets or transferring budgets from one agency to another to run a joint service can seem a threatening proposition. It takes courage and imagination to delegate authority over internal resources to another agency, and there is little political support in local authorities to do this, as it takes decision-making further away from elected councillors and can encourage the growth of powerful officer cliques. Managers also fear that pooling budgets will let the other side realise that they've been paying for things they shouldn't have been all these years!

Working together has to start at the top. In this, there are some rules to be followed. Directors and chief executives across the key agencies must meet regularly with each other to thrash out strategic and operational issues. It is fashionable these days to suggest senior managers in local authorities shouldn't get bogged down in operational matters and should concentrate solely on strategy, but if they don't deal with the most important operational issues, they won't be taken seriously on the wider inter-agency scene, where all other senior managers have to work at both levels. Senior officers must not send substitutes to their meetings with each other, otherwise as time goes by meetings get attended by more and more junior officers who are not authorised to make decisions and are basically note-takers. The process then falls into disrepute.

Working relationships across agencies can be good at the top and terrible at the bottom, or the other way round. Conflicts within agencies can be as great as conflict between agencies. Staff on the ground can be dyed in the wool and resistant to change. The flashier their managers, the more they dig their heels in, however much their managers moan about them. Most professional groups tend to emphasise the importance of what they do, and to understate the contribution of others, or else they see closer working with other professionals potentially threatening their jobs. Each person's separate contribution has to be appreciated and staff need to be able to see, beyond cynicism, how closer working can add to the overall strength of the service. However, most staff are understandably preoccupied with what change means for them as individuals, and not its wider significance.

On the ground, there are clear signs of more inter-agency co-operation. In South Bedfordshire, social services staff and health staff are using common paperwork and information systems to provide joint home care and district nursing services. In many areas, joint provision has been established between district nursing and home care, with joint teams operating, and clear protocols about which skills are needed in which situation. Many basic services require the input and co-operation of a number of agencies and teams in a flowing sequence. For instance, a successful planned hospital discharge of a patient with complex needs will require an accurate diagnosis by a clinician at the hospital and a holistic assessment by a social worker as well as a doctor or nurse of the social and medical support needed at home. Other specialists in hospital such as a physiotherapist may need to assess for the rehabilitation service required at home. An occupational therapist and housing officer, and perhaps a surveyor as well, may need to determine how a property needs a minor adaptation in order for the patient to be able to cope at home with reduced physical abilities or increased frailty. A builder then has to turn up and complete the adaptation job competently. A care manager in the community may need to co-ordinate a range of community care services like home care, respite care and district nursing, also establishing good communication with relatives, within a day or two of the patient being at home; and the patient's GP will need to be made aware of the patient's situation and needs, and to establish a visiting pattern. A single community care process such as this requires the co-ordinated input of a great number of people. If one person's input is missing, it can result in either an unnecessary delay in discharge, or a breakdown of care in the community resulting in a re-admission to hospital. Shortages of resources at any point in the system can also add to the potential hazards at any stage of the process. Similarly, for a young person truanting from school, the active input of an education welfare officer, the school, a social worker, and possibly an outreach youth worker, the police and a youth justice worker, may all be needed to work intensively with the young person during a critical period of days or weeks. If co-ordinated instant support is not put in place, he or she may leave the school system altogether. Getting a young person back to school is always harder than keeping them there in the first place.

## EXAMPLES OF INTER-AGENCY WORKING

### Police and social services joint working

The police have as many operational difficulties as social services. Sometimes local police will not be told of regional drugs squad operations in their area. Some custody officers, faced with young people marooned in custody who shouldn't be there, grow impatient with social workers who won't come and take the young person away. Misunderstandings do arise. When the police ask for a young person to be taken into secure accommodation, they tend to mean simply to a secure location from which he or she can be brought to court when they're due. Social workers take the request for secure accommodation literally, and say either that there aren't any places or that the young person in question doesn't satisfy the criteria. The custody officer then becomes irate. On the other side, social workers become frustrated with the police not being able to arrest and charge many people they deal with who are nasty pieces of work, such as violent partners or service users who intimidate staff repeatedly. Unwillingness to take action on the police's part is more often than not simply a reflection of the limitation of the law.

The current relationship between the police and social services illustrates how inter-agency working is also a function of broader factors in society. Indeed, in the world of inter-agency collaboration, the police and social services are probably the strangest bedfellows of all. In their left-wing heyday, many councils broke off relations with the police altogether. Nowadays they're hardly ever apart. Councils need the police to show they take residents' issues like crime and the fear of crime seriously. The police need councils because they know that most of the people they deal with need a whole range of services that only councils can provide. This marriage of convenience is working quite well. There are one or two hiccups, usually personality-dominated, but current levels of co-operation over youth crime, child protection, risks to elderly people, domestic violence, missing persons and mental health issues would have been unheard of ten years ago. A lot of successful inter-agency work stems purely from confidence-building.

### Schools and social services joint working

The working relationship between schools and social services is frequently stormy. Headteachers and form teachers have insufficient time for pastoral care on top of their other duties, yet they see caring for the wider needs of pupils as part of their job, and part of helping children to capitalise on educational opportunities which they can't possibly take if life at home is in a mess. They would often like social services to do more for the children they're worried about. Pressure of work, or defining priorities differently at the social services end, means schools are often disappointed. They can't understand how some of the children they know, who may have chronic anorexia or bulimia, or who may regularly harm themselves, or who may have stalked teachers and other children issuing serious threats, fail to attract sufficient priority for help. Courts back up the general view in society that a higher level of intervention all round is needed in the lives of children in need. In 1996, in a case of *Re:C* (a minor), a 16-year-old girl with anorexia nervosa was ordered by the High Court to be detained against her will for the purpose of treating her eating disorder.

Welfare support in schools has been decimated by cuts in recent years. Services like education social work are thin on the ground, and the time of back-up staff like educational psychologists tends to go into the statementing process (the formal assessment to determine what additional educational input a child with special educational needs should receive), battling to secure extra tuition or support in class for individual children with emotional, cognitive or behavioural difficulties. Less support for schools within the local education authority infrastructure drives them to seek more from social services.

Another battleground where regular skirmishing takes place is the transmission of information. Schools complain social workers never tell them anything, including when children come into care and are suddenly living with foster carers. Social workers think the concerns about children passed over by schools have to be discussed with the child's parents, which is basically right unless disclosing the information would result in the child being directly harmed as a result. Schools then often blame social workers for breaking a confidence and damaging their relationship with a parent who may not tell them, they worry, anything else. These are bread and butter issues which staff from both sides have to be clear about in relation to each individual case. A general rule isn't going to be of much use. The pressures of daily working lives militate against effective communication. The teacher tries to call the social worker in between lessons. The social worker's on another line, and so on. Finding time to communicate properly is the key. Meeting face to face to iron out disagreements and seek a way of resolving conflicts and moving forward with a jointly agreed plan can avert months of niggles.

### Carol's story

Carol is the head teacher at a suburban junior school. Tom was a colleague, a fellow teacher for several years. They were both in a holiday hotel with other teachers and children when Alan, a 10-year-old boy, told Carol he didn't like the way Tom touched him. Carol immediately sent Tom home while Alan's allegation could be investigated. Both Alan and his parents wanted the holiday to continue, but the holiday was understandably a troubled one for

Carol and Alan. Alan's request to Carol was simple: 'I want you to stop it happening'. Carol made copious notes at the time, which were to prove a great help later.

The investigation revealed a long history of concern about Tom, who outside school was also working with children. Tom, according to a number of children interviewed, massaged boys' legs – his victims were always boys – played rough games with them, insisted they weren't to wear underpants, and pulled their shorts down. Once the concerns about Tom became public knowledge, some parents, including parents of boys in the town where he lived, said they had always been worried about him, and wouldn't let their own sons attend any activity he ran or organised. A few years before, one complaint had been made to the local social services team in his local area, but this was not acted upon.

A few months later, Tom was charged at the local Crown Court with indecent assault on a number of boys. More than ten children had made separate statements as part of a police and social services investigation. It was clear that the children, who were of different ages and in unrelated friendship groups, could not be part of a conspiracy. Tom denied all the charges. Carol had to hold the school together in the meantime, and reassure everyone, teachers, pupils and parents alike. Both teachers and children were at times distressed. The children who were due to give evidence were well supported by a specialist witness support police officer, and the teachers were helped by the school's educational psychologist who often came down at a moment's notice. In fact, all the professionals acted more than competently, and the tense situation was well handled. The detective from the police child protection team was sensitive to what everyone was going through. The local social work manager chaired a series of strategy discussions expertly. Carol and the other staff directly involved formed a small support network for each other. The school governors and parents were highly supportive, and through this the school gained greater strength as a community.

At the trial, Tom's barrister tried to tie both adult and child witnesses up in knots, seeking to discredit their reliability. He intimidated them, and this was compounded by the judge eventually implying to the jury that what Tom did was not too serious. The jury found him not guilty inside half an hour, finding the case was not proven beyond reasonable doubt.

Tom was sacked at an internal disciplinary hearing, as the basis of the finding was on the less strict 'balance of probabilities' rule. He continued to work with children but not as a teacher. It is not inconceivable that he will surface again as a teacher in another part of the country in the future. After it was all over, Carol sent all the staff on child protection training. She still has nightmares and flashbacks about what happened. So do some of the children, whose behaviour is less confident as a result of the episode, perhaps because in the most formal setting they had ever been, a British Crown Court, they were not taken seriously. From start to finish, these events took over two years to resolve, although in many ways it is still far from over.

These examples show how working across agencies is far from straightforward, but that when it works well, it has a multiplier effect on confidence. To some extent, the world of welfare has become so fragmented, because of political changes like the internal health market, local management of schools, and GP commissioning, that the centre of the welfare system, to paraphrase W.B. Yeats, cannot longer hold. Mirroring the shift in British society from subject to citizen status, the world of social care professionals is now a hard one to chart, with so many different individuals and groups with something to say and something to contribute. Pluralism has its dangers. Just as it can lead to wider and deeper consultation and involvement, it can also lead the people at the very top of the tree to consolidate their own power because opposition is everywhere and nowhere simultaneously. This is especially true when unwieldy bureaucratic structures are dismantled. Often the benefits of linear bureaucracies, such as their formal systems of accountability and their visible political process, are only appreciated when they are gone and the new looser arrangements that have taken their place, like management boards for inter-agency community care services who rarely see the need to meet, are harder for stakeholders like staff and voluntary sector organisations to understand and influence. Taking the politics out of politics may unwittingly create the public sector equivalent of Frankenstein's monster.

# Chapter 13

# Across the borders
## Scotland and Northern Ireland

There may be no passport controls for those who journey to Scotland or Northern Ireland from elsewhere in the UK but to visit those places is to cross a legislative and administrative divide.

Wales and England (though the former has its own Secretary of State and government department and will have its own assembly – see below) share legal systems. There are only two ways in which Wales differs administratively at the moment from England and these are marginal. The first is that its local government structure (introduced in April 1996) is slightly different from that of its neighbour. It formerly enjoyed a two-tier system of local government, in which the eight county councils provided social services. With the abolition of the counties (and the thirty-seven district councils) in April 1996 it joined Scotland in having only one level of local government with twenty-two unitary authorities. England's social services are shared between counties, some district councils and thirty-two London boroughs.

The second difference concerns only one service – for people with learning difficulties – but it is an example often pointed to because of its uniqueness and progressive nature. The All-Wales Mental Handicap (now Learning Difficulties) Strategy is a unique approach which combines specially earmarked money and, critically, the decision that central government (Welsh Office) should take a directive lead in the way in which services would be run (Philpot 1993).

Scotland's systems and practice, often seen as being in advance of the rest of the UK, have developed from its different history. Northern Ireland's structures arose largely from the civil and political unrest of the late 1960s.

## SCOTLAND

As has often been the case, Scotland's social work reforms preceded those south of the border. The Social Work (Scotland) Act was passed in 1968 as the Seebohm Committee was being set up in England and Wales (see Chapter 1). Thus, Scotland was the first place in the UK to offer a comprehensive welfare service. As long ago as 1963, the McBoyle Committee on child neglect (McBoyle 1963) had recommended a comprehensive family service. Hand in hand with a comprehensive approach were the reforms in dealing with juvenile offenders – the creation of the children's hearing system, with panels rather than courts. But while in England and Wales the Seebohm reform of social services came two years before the local government landscape was redrawn (see Chapter 1), Scotland waited until 1975 for its new authorities, the regional councils, to be created.

The new Scottish local government system – powerful regions that ran the social work service, sitting above district councils – was suited to the ambitions of its social services reforms. Regions were very much what the name implies. England and Wales had counties, only some of which, at that time, were social services authorities. Scotland's regions mostly covered very large areas; indeed, Strathclyde, which took in the islands of the former Hebrides as well as Glasgow, could claim to be the largest local authority in Europe.

The primacy of social work as a profession in Scotland was shown by the use of the term 'social work' when describing reforms and services and as part of the title of departments. In England, Wales and Northern Ireland the term 'social services' is most commonly used, partly to reflect the fact that social workers constitute only a minority of the workforce in social services departments, and also as an umbrella term to include social work, residential and day care, occupational therapy and the home help (domiciliary) care services, all of which, as also in Scotland, come under social services departments.

The new Scottish social work departments came out of a three-person advisory group – Richard Titmuss, Kay Carmichael and Megan Browne – appointed by the Secretary of State for Scotland. Previous suggestions had not envisaged what were to become the powerful, all-embracing social work departments. In 1964 the Kilbrandon Committee (Kilbrandon 1964) had suggested that education departments should be responsible for social work services. This would have made social work a secondary activity in departments whose primary purpose and function would have been education. But the Secretary of State's group drew together a coalition of social work, civil service and political interests. Judith Hart, the then Under-Secretary of State for Scotland, who favoured social work, also played a critical role in the outcome. All this led directly to the White Paper of 1966, *Social Work and the Community* (Scottish Education and Scottish Home and Health Departments 1966), which in turn led to the Social Work (Scotland) Act.

While in England and Wales the Seebohm Committee had acknowledged the role of social work, the Scottish White Paper proposed that the new departments would be 'based on the insights and skills of the profession of social work'. One commentator stated:

> The use of the term 'social work' in this legislation was symbolic of the largely successful struggle by social work interests in Scotland to use the opportunity provided by the initial concern to make effective provision for dealing with delinquency [the Kilbrandon recommendations]. This was the jumping-off point for a comprehensive social work service enabling social work to achieve parity with education and health departments.
>
> (Adams 1996)

Not only were social work departments to be their own masters and housed within the regions but the reforms were more inclusive than the Seebohm changes. The school welfare service and child guidance (although educational psychologists were employed by education departments), as well as the probation service and the prison social work service, came under the social work departments.

More importantly, the departments had an extraordinary legal duty laid upon them by the Act which did not apply elsewhere in the UK: this was 'to promote social welfare by making available advice, guidance and assistance on such a scale as may be appropriate for their areas' (Section 12). The section goes on to state that help in 'kind and cash' may be given to individuals in certain circumstances.

The new departments would work flexibly but specialisms would continue to be practised. Not only would social work departments plan services to meet the distinct needs of communities but they would also advise other local authority departments about the impact of those departments' policies on communities and individuals. Scottish local authority social work has always been stronger in the fields of community work and community development than England and Wales. This stems partly from a more collective national ethos but also from the emphasis on general planning by the new departments, tailoring services to meet the community's needs, and the duty to promote the welfare of communities and individuals. The departments also pioneered the development of welfare rights for many of the same reasons.

But in April 1996 the twelve regional and island authorities and the fifty-three district (non-social services) authorities were abolished and a single-tier system of thirty-two district authorities, responsible for social work, as well as housing and education and other services, was created. Unlike in England and Wales, where commissions were established to look at local situations and make recommendations to the Secretaries of State, some of which were implemented and some not, in Scotland the map of local government was rewritten by ministerial fiat.

For social work there were other important considerations. Despite a great deal of lobbying by various bodies and professional associations, the government refused to make it a statutory requirement that each local authority should not only have to appoint a director of social work but that person would have to be someone who held a social work qualification. This double requirement, which existed in Scotland up to the 1996 reorganisation, did not apply elsewhere. It was a formal affirmation of the status of social work and its values. Most local authorities did appoint a chief officer with the title of director of social work and most of them held a social work qualification. However, some authorities appointed a chief social work officer who was responsible to a chief officer who headed an omnibus department, the responsibilities of which might combine, say, housing and social work and even, in some cases, leisure services. Where this happened, this was seen as a downgrading of the status of social work.

This seemed to combine insult and injury to a social work profession reared in the halcyon days of 1968. Despite funding problems which affected social services throughout the UK (although Scotland has received significantly 19 per cent above the UK average for health and personal social services (Department of Finance and Personnel 1997)), there had been twenty-five years of solid achievement. Significantly and notwithstanding the events in

Orkney and Ayr, Scotland has been remarkably free of 'child abuse scandals' which had so sapped the self-confidence of English social work. Whether the loss of the powerful regions combined with a lower status for social work services will threaten the very existence of social work as so many Scottish Jeremiahs suggest will not be known for some while. The new authorities, created in April 1996, found themselves facing a crisis brought on by spending cuts introduced by the then government. But even if the death of social work was an exaggeration, a lack of confidence about its resilience and political support had at last spread north of the border.

Scotland's pioneering approach to dealing with young offenders was unaffected by local government reorganisation. In England and Wales, eighteen years of Conservative government overturned 1960s' notions of welfare rather than punishment for this group of young people, something which was enthusiastically taken up by the Labour Government. But perhaps it is significant that there were no governmental calls in Scotland to move away from what was the most welfare-orientated system for young offenders in the UK.

Children's hearings are independent bodies but they arose from the Kilbrandon Report which had favoured a comprehensive family service, albeit one it envisaged in a social education department. They were created under the Social Work (Scotland) Act 1968. The Kilbrandon Committee had been set up at a time of concern over rising juvenile crime rates. It began very much from scratch: juvenile courts were by no means as universal in Scotland as they were in England. Kilbrandon's thinking chimed very much with the contemporary 'treatment as opposed to punishment' approach to dealing with young offenders, which was evidenced in the Children and Young Persons Act 1969 for England and Wales. The committee saw little difference between children who came before the courts and those who were in need of care, protection or control. In essence, it saw criminality as related to deprivation of various kinds. The report opined: 'The shortcomings inherent in the juvenile court system can . . . be traced essentially to the fact that they are required to combine the characteristics of a court of law with those of a specialised agency for the treatment of children in need' (Kilbrandon 1964).

The hearings or panels consist of a group of trained lay people (a panel). Hearings are not courts of law. They deal with children and young people aged 8 to 16, which are the ages of criminal responsibility for Scottish children (it is 10 to 17 in England and

Wales). The onset of criminal responsibility at 8 in Scotland is in rather stark contrast to generally liberal Scottish methods of dealing with young offenders.

If the child or young person admits an offence, is found guilty of one before a sheriff's (magistrate's) court and appears to need 'compulsory measures of care' (Section 39), or may be subject to ill treatment or is not attending school, the case is referred to an independent official, the reporter. Reporters were created by the Act, are appointed by local authorities but cannot be removed without the consent of the Secretary of State. Referrals can be made by anyone but most are made by social workers. The reporter investigates and decides either to take no action, or to refer the case to the social work department, or if, as Section 39 of the Act puts it, 'it appears to the reporter that the child is in need of compulsory measures of care he [the reporter] shall arrange a children's hearing'. At the hearing the child (or its parents) either accepts or denies the grounds for the referral (this may be admitting an offence). If they do not, then it goes to the sheriff who decides. If the sheriff decides that the grounds are established then the case goes back to the hearing. Then panel members receive reports from social workers, listen to the child and parents before deciding what should happen to the child. (Certain offences, such as murder and rape, cannot be dealt with by the hearings.)

Hearings have wide discretion to deal with offenders. They do so usually with child and parents present. Their role is to decide what non-punitive sentences would be appropriate. The hearing can impose a supervision order, which can include the child going into some kind of residential care. The panel continues an interest in the case with (if appropriate) annual reviews. The panel can vary or terminate orders, according to an offender's progress. It cannot impose punitive sentences. It cannot, for example, fine the child or the parents or send the case to the sheriff for sentence.

For a quarter of a century progressive English eyes have looked longingly at the hearings system. Such feelings have not been especially mitigated by the creation, in England and Wales, by the Criminal Justice Act 1991, of the youth court, which has taken over the criminal proceedings aspects of the now-defunct juvenile court. In the youth courts, as in the hearings, proceedings tend to be more informal than in other types of court. The public are excluded and the press are not allowed to identify those appearing before the court or hearing.

Scotland had to wait six years after the Children Act 1989 had been passed for England and Wales for its own reformed child care legislation in the shape of the Children (Scotland) Act 1995. But as with other Scottish legislation its genesis was different from that elsewhere. It arose from many sources – numerous reports, the Scottish Child Care Review (Scottish Office 1990), as well as the events in Orkney (Clyde 1992) and Fife (Kearney 1992).

There are similarities between the Children (Scotland) Act and the Children Act. Notably, both are underpinned by the principle that the welfare of the child must be paramount in any decision taken by the courts. The two pieces of legislation are similar also in many details, such as the duty of local authorities to publish children's plans (though in Scotland the responsibility rests with the chief executive), and place of safety orders being replaced by child protection and child assessment orders (the child protection orders make the criteria for removing a child from its home more stringent). Parental responsibilities can only be granted by a court order. Local authorities are also under a duty to consider a child's religious persuasion, racial origin and cultural and linguistic background when placing them for adoption. 'Custody' and 'access' were replaced by 'residence' and 'contact'. Children are no longer 'in care' of the local authority but 'looked after' by it. This new term encompasses all children living in residential homes, or who are fostered or who live at home under supervision orders imposed by the hearings, and those subject to child protection orders. Like the Children Act, the Scottish legislation balances parental rights with parental responsibilities. There is also a new procedure for unmarried fathers to obtain parental rights with the agreement of the mother.

As with the Children Act, local authorities are also given a duty (not a discretion, as in England and Wales) to help 'children in need'. But in Scotland the concept differs slightly in that children affected by the disability of another family member are included as well as children who are themselves disabled. Local authorities' duty to assist young people leaving care is extended to the 19th birthday, with a discretion to assist up to the age of 21.

But there are also significant differences. Scotland now has exclusion orders which mean that a court can order someone alleged to have committed child abuse to be removed from the home where the child is living. Sheriffs can grant child protection orders and exclusion orders to force those guilty of abuse to be excluded from the family home, and can also supervise the continuing role of the children's hearings in these matters. The hearings have the power to exclude parents, other individuals and the press to allow a child to speak more freely. (But anyone excluded has the right to be told the substance of what was said in their absence.) Sheriffs are now allowed to hear new evidence on the grounds of referral to a hearing and the rights of appeal for children and parents have been extended. There is some concern, though, that in considering an appeal a sheriff may substitute his or her own decision for that of a hearing. Hearings also have had the grounds for referral altered (these now include drug misuse).

Community care was slower in coming to Scotland than England and Wales and the development of a mixed economy of care, with a split between purchasers and providers, which underpins community care, was even slower. Progress on the reforms in Scotland, with their attendant increased role for the voluntary and private sectors, may also have lagged behind because of a greater belief in public provision by Scottish directors than their English and Welsh counterparts, who enthusiastically embraced the reforms almost as soon as they were announced. But there is in Scotland, arguably, a greater trust by the public of social services and the Scots have had also perhaps less cause to mistrust such services.

Scotland will have a parliament from 2000. In both Scotland and Wales, local authorities will continue to be responsible for social services. The only service with which social work is concerned and which will be devolved is the NHS. What impact, if any, this will have on social work is impossible to predict at this stage.

The Scottish Parliament, unlike the assembly in Wales, will have 'tax-varying' powers, that is, it will be able to raise or lower the standard rate of income tax. No guess can be made at the implications of the ability of the Scottish Parliament to 'vary' income tax – given the Scots' favour of public services and public spending it is not difficult to imagine that any variation upwards might benefit social services. But this could be minimal in that the 'variation' could account for only £450 million compared with the present (1997) Scottish Office block grant of £14 billion which Westminster allocates to Scotland.

The new governments for Scotland and Wales will inherit the Secretaries of States' powers to issue guidance and direction to social services and social work departments. This could affect issues as fundamental as charging for services, working between different agencies in the care of people with a mental illness, or the balance between family support and child protection services. In the former case of charging, it may iron out inconsistencies between different departments as there is a great variation at the moment between policies in one area and policies in another. But a more uniform approach need not have waited on devolution – Whitehall is quite able to issue guidance to deal with inconsistencies. The parliament and assembly will also be able to ask the Westminster Parliament to review legislation where they believe it inappropriate to their countries.

## NORTHERN IRELAND

Northern Ireland's history of sectarian strife and political turbulence has left more than a deep mark on its administrative structure: it has shaped it. Indeed, one of the reasons for the rise of the civil rights movement in the 1960s was the demand for the reform of local government. It was felt to be subject to gerrymandering and corruption, a locus of Protestant dominance and political manipulation and, consequently, was a deep-seated source of Catholic dissatisfaction. It was also the case that, while as Adams (1996) correctly argues, radical change was brought about by political imperatives, local government, as then constituted, was inadequate to its task of service provision (Cooper 1983). The end result was a unified health and social services structure accountable to Westminster through the Northern Ireland civil service and Secretary of State.

As long ago as 1947 the Welfare Services Act established local authority education and public health and services for children and elderly people. The following year legislation had made hospitals responsible for the care of mentally ill people, and in 1950 each local authority was required by law to set up a welfare department for elderly and disabled people and children.

In August 1969 the British government sent troops into Northern Ireland, initially welcomed by the Catholic population, who saw the Army as their protectors against their Protestant Unionist oppressors. But this turned to hardened opposition on the part of Catholics, who came to see the Army as an occupying force supporting the oppressor.

However, at the same time as the government was using military means to deal with the situation, it hoped to effect a political solution. Three months after troops arrived a review of local government was announced which was chaired by Patrick Macrory. The intention was to see how local government's responsibilities could be more efficiently shared between the Westminster government and the one then existing in Northern Ireland. The old Stormont government had administered (among other services) health and social services.

Not charged with having to consider local democracy in what it suggested, Macrory's recommendations became law in 1972. The number of district councils (for a population of 1.5 million) was cut from sixty-eight to twenty-six and nine area boards were set up to take over the provision of health, education and social services.

But the same year as the Local Government (NI) Act set up the new system, the Health and Social Services (Northern Ireland) Order refined it further and established four boards – the Northern, Eastern, Southern and Western – to co-ordinate health and social care provision. The health and social services boards, whose members are directly appointed by ministers, have given Northern Ireland what many regard as an advantage over the rest of the UK – the NHS and social services are provided under one administrative roof. However, more than elsewhere in the UK the lack of professionally qualified staff for many years hampered service development. It is also a cause of disquiet for some that while the boards are responsible for the largest amount of public social spending on two of the most critical services, they are not democratically elected. In this respect, boards are the same as the boards of NHS trusts. Thus, they differ markedly from social work and social services elsewhere in the UK, where those services are a part of democratically elected local government. (Housing and probation are also run by two separate province-wide quangos, the Northern Ireland Housing Executive and the Northern Ireland Probation Board, the members of both of which are also appointed by ministers.)

It is also arguable that social work and social services in Northern Ireland have lost status by reforms which succeeded those of the early 1970s. In 1983 the first Griffiths Report (as opposed to that which ushered in the community care reforms) on health service management recommended a new general management structure for the NHS (Griffiths 1983). However, the government decided to apply this to Northern Ireland on the grounds that the NHS there was managed within the unified boards (Philpot 1985). Thus, general managers appointed to head the boards supplanted the directors of social services' chief officer status. But worse was to come: later reforms, developed from the principles of general management, ended directors of social services' role as operational managers, essentially reducing them to advisers.

The health and social services boards exist within a governmental structure where the quango has been given full rein. In a province with a population of only 1.6 million, there are twenty-six district councils, four health and social services boards, five education boards, a probation board, a training and employment agency, twenty-one health and social services trusts and a housing executive – many of them with regional offices – not to mention six government departments. And, increasingly, there is the European Union, whose massive funding of work in Northern Ireland has given a critical role to the voluntary sector as a channel for funds.

Northern Ireland's unified health and social services are not the province's only administrative peculiarity. Elsewhere in the UK, the purchaser/provider split in social services (see Chapters 2, 3, 5 and 6) is predicated on the local authority purchasing and commissioning services from the voluntary and private sectors. In Northern Ireland the boards were encouraged to cease to provide any services and, under the Health and Personal Social Services Orders of 1991 and 1994, 'units of management' – the lowest rung of administration which has traditionally provided services – could become self-governing trusts, legally separate from the boards. The boards, then, are the purchasers and the health and social services trusts are, save for a few exceptions, the providers, and may, if they wish, subcontract for services, but are not required to do so. (The orders did not permit boards to carry out statutory child care functions. But the 1994 Order allowed boards to delegate such work to trusts.) By the end of April 1996 there were eleven trusts providing personal social services. Some also provided community and acute hospital services and other only social care and community health. Again, as with the introduction of general management, the system has followed the NHS (health as opposed to social services) model where providers are mostly in the public sector (the so-called 'internal market').

While Northern Ireland's unified health and social services system is an advantage over the bipartite structures elsewhere, the country, like Scotland, also enjoys a strong tradition of community work (one strengthened by the Troubles), albeit mainly in the voluntary sector, as well as having a long history of voluntary sector work, partly through the strength of the churches and also through the long-established voluntary agencies. In a population of 1.6 million there are an estimated 5,300 voluntary bodies, with an annual turnover of £400 million – equal to 6 per cent of Northern Ireland's GDP – and assets of £250 million. There are 65,000 volunteers in a sector which employs 30,000 paid workers – or 5 per cent of the workforce, more than those employed in agriculture (Northern Ireland Council for Voluntary Action 1997).

One consequence of the last twenty-five years has been that with a virtually powerless local government and effective power resting with Westminster, the voluntary sector has stepped into the democratic vacuum and become the locus of civil society. Its importance gained official sanction and recognition in 1993 when the government and the sector (represented by the Northern Ireland Council for Voluntary Action) agreed a 'support strategy' (Philpot 1997).

The strategy document (Northern Ireland Office 1993) 'acknowledges the role and contribution to many aspects of life in Northern Ireland' of the sector and then lays down guidelines for good practice for all government departments 'through common and agreed principles'. Some of the points which it makes are unremarkable but there are four which do mark a significant step forward in how government, in Northern Ireland at least, views the voluntary sector. First, the strategy document sees the sector as involved not only in providing services but formally recognises its role in making policy. Second, it says that all departments should consider the impact on the sector of new and existing policies. Third, it gives the sector the right to be consulted on proposed changes which might affect it. Fourth, community development – as in Scotland, a stronger force in Northern Ireland than in England and Wales – is also given recognition.

Northern Ireland's child care law, like that in England and Wales and in Scotland, underwent a radical reform with the passing in 1995 of the Children (Northern Ireland) Order. This was modelled on the Children Act more closely than was the Children (Scotland) Act and its differences, where they exist, very largely reflect the difference between the organisation of health and social services in Northern Ireland and England and Wales.

Like the Children Act, the order is based on the principle of promoting the children's welfare, seeking to strike a balance between the rights of children to be consulted, the rights of parents in exercising their responsibilities towards their children and the right of the state to intervene to protect or promote the welfare of children 'in need' or at risk.

One major difference between the order and the Act is that the former had to allow for the creation of a guardian *ad litem* system, which previously did not exist in Northern Ireland. (Guardians are independent social workers, selected from a panel, who provide social work opinions to a court about what is best for a child's welfare in civil proceedings like adoption, care proceedings and child protection.)

The order also lowered the age from 14 to 13 under which employing children is prohibited and also removed an earlier (1968) prohibition on the employment of children for more than two hours on a Sunday. Under the order also no children's homes were exempted from registration, whereas under the Act only those providing for more than three children at any one time needed to be registered. The definition of 'disabled', said to be demeaning to disabled children, was not altered in the consultation period and there was no definition in the order of what constitutes a child 'in need'.

Two other major changes came with the order. Only one of the province's four training schools for young offenders (although most of the young people accommodated were there as a result of care orders – equivalent to the old approved schools in England) remained unchanged. Three of them ceased to be training schools, two becoming voluntary sector children's homes (they were run by the Catholic Church) and the other a statutory children's home.

The second other major change caused by the order was that the amount of secure accommodation – residential care with locked doors and windows and restricted movement within and outside the premises – was greatly reduced as the order did not permit such accommodation to be run by voluntary sector child care organisations. By contrast, in England and Wales at about the same time the government was inviting voluntary child care agencies to provide more secure accommodation to meet a national shortage.

The 1998 Northern Ireland Agreement, if it holds, will lead to a new model of local government in the province, with potential implications for the organisation and delivery of social services. Indeed, increasing devolution in Scotland, Wales and Northern Ireland may bring in much greater regional variations in social care, policy and practice.

# Chapter 14

# Conclusion
## Into the future

Social work and social care services approach the millennium with uncertainty and anxiety as their companions. It is not, as we have sought to show, that there is not a demonstrable necessity for such services. But the broad picture, which we have also tried to paint, is that these vital services are stretched to the limit by pressure on resources, staff limitations and a lack of public and political sympathy, allied with serious and (in some cases) long-standing deficiencies in services which social services departments have failed to remedy.

There is something of a rhetorical gap between statements about services as articulated in the business plans, children's services plans and community care plans of local authorities (and, indeed, those statements made by voluntary organisations about their intentions) and what the public sometimes receives. Yet social services are being positively influenced by the corporate direction taken by local authorities and, despite well-publicised shortcomings, moves towards greater collaboration with other agencies, like health and housing. However, whatever fears social services departments and social workers have about their own future, the outlook for those who use services must be immeasurably more problematic.

It would be complacent to claim that all would be well with social services if only there were more money to offer more of the same. Our contention has been that while resources are often scarce, the organisation and delivery of care services remain a problem. It is wrong to talk about one without the other, wrong to blame resource shortfalls for everything, but equally wrong not to point out how resource constraints add to the social stresses and failures in services we have described. Three official reports published in 1997 indicate just how far some services fall short of an acceptable standard and thus why change is necessary. The annual report of Sir Herbert Laming, Chief Inspector of social services, identified major gaps in the service nationally, including poor case recording, management information systems and care planning (Laming 1997). All of these are essential components of first-class social services.

A Social Services Inspectorate report on services for deaf and hard of hearing people found that 'the quality and extent of services across the authorities [inspected] was disappointing with only one [out of eight] presenting a generally satisfactory picture' (Social Services Inspectorate 1997a). Inspectors found the situation little better and, in some respects, probably worse, than the services provided by the pre-Seebohm welfare departments in the 1960s. As up to 8.5 million people in the UK experience profound hearing loss, the whole area of sensory disability remains a neglected one, requiring major developments in services.

A third report, also by the Social Services Inspectorate, into services provided for adopted children and their adoptive families, was similarly critical (Social Services Inspectorate 1997b).

We have referred earlier to the reams of guidance on practice and management issued by government, notably that arising from the Children Act and the NHS and Community Care Act, and in particular, with regard to the former legislation, *Working Together* (Department of Health 1991) and *Child Protection: Messages from Research* (Department of Health 1995). There has also been in the 1990s a clearer framework of legislation, as well as guidance. Despite this, there is ample evidence that guidance is not followed and lessons are not learned. Sometimes this results in bad practice but 1997 was notable for the publication of two reports which found that front-line staff were not coping against the odds partly created by the serious deficiencies of management. The Social Services Inspectorate and the Audit Commission found that in Sefton, Merseyside, almost 200 children needing help and protection had not been allocated a social worker (Social Services Inspectorate/ Audit Commission 1997a). The inspectorate's report into child protection services in Cambridgeshire (Social Services Inspectorate 1997c) found a lack of action two years after the death of 6-year-old Rikki Neave, the event which had prompted the report. The Chief Inspector, Sir Herbert Laming, went so far as to say: 'At this time, I cannot be confident that children at risk in the county are safe from significant harm or neglect.' He went on to blame management for frustrating front-line staff by 'an absence of direction, effective procedures and inefficient management' (quoted in Cresswell 1997).

One of the seemingly intractable problems in child protection work was identified by Allan Levy QC, who himself co-chaired the inquiry into 'pin-down' in Staffordshire in 1990–91, when he succinctly summed up the situation after the Cambridgeshire report appeared. He said:

> There have been at least 30 significant inquiries in the last 20 years, if not more. It is the same scenario over and over again and it has been going on for years. We are just not following up on these recommendations [in the inquiry reports]. When you look through the various reports you are reading the same material, the same recommendations, the same failings.
>
> (quoted in Castle and Dobson 1997)

We have also drawn attention to inconsistencies in services across the country, both in the volume of services provided, resource levels, and in other ways, such as the number of children placed on child protection registers. These variations are far greater than can be explained by differences in local needs or even spending patterns. The joint reviews of social services departments, undertaken by the Department of Health and the Audit Commission, have also shown considerable differences in performance from authority to authority. These are failures of national policies, not just of individual organisations.

The challenge to improve the standards of care is one of the greatest which faces health and social services. In a psychiatric hospital close to where one of the authors works, the night shift on one particular ward put elderly patients to bed by restraining them in drawer sheets so that they couldn't move. Down the road, at a hostel for people with learning difficulties, a culture of mimicking and undermining service users was uncovered by a whistleblower. Both incidents took place late in 1997. These are but two anecdotes known to the authors. There are others which attest to abuse, humiliation, petty cruelty and simple carelessness which leads to serious injury or even death, some of which are recorded in this book and others of which are found in each day's newspapers. The need for change extends to attitude. In a nearby day centre to the psychiatric hospital mentioned above, people with physical disabilities being taken on an outing are still being referred to as 'walkers, feeders and chairs', rather than Bill, Tom, Irene and Jane.

No amount of reorganisation (one of the continuing non-solutions to problems beloved of governments and individual local authorities for the past twenty-five years) or business planning meetings can right the wrongs noted above. True, paedophiles and abusers of different kinds have infiltrated services, in particular residential care services. But the shortcomings of practice cannot all be put down to those who enter services so that they have access to vulnerable people, serious though this problem is. For the rest, there are shortages of people like nurses and occupational therapists. Residential social work, in particular, suffers from the combined disadvantages of low public esteem, low pay, poor conditions and a majority of untrained staff, whether at managerial or worker level. Social workers still do not enjoy the 3-year qualifying training which is common in the majority of other EU countries. Together such factors encourage employers to take the risk of employing unqualified and untrained people and put a greater reliance on private personnel and care agencies, where recruitment standards are mixed and whose staff, no matter how well motivated or qualified, cannot be expected to offer the commitment and continuity so essential for those with whom they will work.

Social services will continue to exist. If they did not, like Voltaire's God, there would be a need to invent them. There is no such guarantee of the ways in which, or the means by which, they will be provided. That they will be increasingly intended for the more vulnerable, as eligibility criteria are tightened, seems inevitable. But alongside the mainstream services, whether provided by the voluntary, statutory or private sectors, other services need to be developed if mainstream services are not to be used to paper over the cracks. These 'new' services include more support for carers, more development and training for volunteers, and more mobile and flexible services that are more responsive to what those who use them want.

Like any ailing industry, social services will need renewal and new investment in the skills base, infrastructure and resources if it is to come of age in the twenty-first century. Yet, despite the problems and acknowledged shortcomings, there is evidence that, while social services come under attack from media and politicians, customer satisfaction is not lacking. For example, the first of the joint reviews, carried out by the Social Services Inspectorate and the

Audit Commission, in Stockport, found that 73 per cent of those who used services were highly satisfied with what they received (Social Services Inspectorate/Audit Commission 1997b).

The intention of this book has been, first, to explain the work of social services and the historical, political, managerial and financial contexts in which they have developed and are provided. But we have also sought to show how critical social services are to welfare. As Britain, like all nations, undergoes rapid technological, social and cultural change, social services provide a safety net, however frayed and worn. They are, as we began by quoting in the foreword, 'the fourth arm of the welfare state', according to the former Conservative Health Secretary Stephen Dorrell. Social services offer an enduring and necessary image and expression of compassion, which stretches from the early work of the philanthropic pioneers to those who, often with small reward and little thanks, today provide and care for the frequently hidden victims of our society.

# Notes

## FOREWORD

1 Wootton, B (1978) 'The social work task today', *Community Care*, 4 October.

## INTRODUCTION

1 *New York Times*, 15 August 1997.

## 2 ON THE STATUTE BOOK

1 P. Marsh and J. Triseliotis (1996) *Ready to Practise? Social Workers and Probation Officers: Their Training and First Year in Practice*, Aldershot: Avebury Press.

2 Joyce Plotnikoff and Richard Woolfson (1996) *Reporting to Court under the Children Act*, London: HMSO.

3 *National Standards for the Supervision of Offenders in the Community* (1995), London: Home Office Publications Unit. Also relevant is the *National Protocol for Youth Justice Services: Statements of Principle for Local Services in England and Wales* (1996), London: Association of Metropolitan Authorities.

4 *Memorandum of Good Practice (on video-recorded interviews with child witnesses for criminal proceedings)* (1992), London: HMSO, followed on by *The Child, the Court and the Video (a study of the implementation of the Memorandum of Good Practice)* (1994), Heywood: Social Services Inspectorate.

5 *Home Life: A Code of Practice for Residential Care* (1984), London: Centre for Policy on Ageing.

6 Alison Taylor (1996) *In Guilty Night*, London: Robert Hale Ltd.

7 *'Whistleblowers': Guidance for Social Services on Free Expression of Staff Concerns* (1995), Birmingham: The British Association of Social Workers (BASW).

8 Brian Littlechild (1996) *The Police and Criminal Evidence Act (1984):*

*The Role of the Appropriate Adult* (revised edition), Birmingham: The British Association of Social Workers (BASW).

9 J. Iqbal (1991) *Report on Ethnic Minority Groups and Occupational Therapy Services in East Birmingham*, Birmingham: City of Birmingham Social Services Department.

## 3 THE NUTS AND BOLTS OF CARE

1 A point well brought out by Gerald Smale (1996) in *Mapping Change and Innovation*, London: HMSO.

2 Terry Bamford (1996) 'Information driven decision-making: fact or fantasy?', in A. Kerslake and N. Gould (eds) *Information Management in Social Services*, Aldershot: Ashgate Publishing.

3 Lesley Hoyes (1996) 'Personal social services for older people', in S. Leach, H. Davis *et al.* (eds) *Enabling or Disabling Local Government*, Milton Keynes: Open University Press.

4 P. Neate (1997) 'The commitments', *Community Care*, 24–30 April.

5 P. Neate (1995) 'In focus', *Community Care*, 9–15 February.

6 P. Marsh and J. Triseliotis (1996) *Ready to Practise? Social Workers and Probation Officers: Their Training and First Year in Practice*, Aldershot: Avebury Press.

## 4 FOR THE CHILD'S SAKE

1 M. Dunn and J. McCluskey (1997) *NCH Action For Children '98 Fact File*, NCH: London.

2 Central Statistical Office (1994) *Social Focus on Children*, London: HMSO.

3 Government Statistical Service, Department of Health (1996) *Children and Young People on Child Protection Register, Year Ending 31 March 1995*, London: HMSO.

4 H. Laming (1997) *Better Management, Better Care: The Sixth Annual Report of the Chief Inspector of Social Services*, London: HMSO.

5 *A Child in Trust: The Report of the Panel of Inquiry into the Circumstances Surrounding the Death of Jasmine Beckford* (1985), London: London Borough of Brent.

6 *Report of the Committee of Inquiry into the Care and Supervision Provided in Relation to Maria Colwell* (1974), London: HMSO.

7 *Whose Child? The Report of the Public Inquiry into the Death of Tyra Henry* (1987), London: London Borough of Lambeth.

8 *A Child in Mind: The Report of the Inquiry into the Circumstances Surrounding the Death of Kimberley Carlile* (1987), London: London Borough of Greenwich.

9 *Report of the Inquiry into Child Abuse in Cleveland* (1988), London: HMSO.

10 For a concise introduction to a number of high-profile child protection cases, including their implications, the reader is advised to go to

P. Reder, S. Duncan and M. Gray (1993) *Beyond Blame*, London: Routledge.

11  Bride Child Care Consultancy (1996) *The Rikki Neave Report*, Cambridge: Cambridgeshire County Council.

12  Case discussed in a conversation with Dr Alison Beck, Clinical Psychologist, Shaftesbury Clinic, Springfield Hospital, Tooting, London.

13  Department of Health statistics, see note 3 (this chapter).

14  *Report of the Panel of Inquiry Presented to Tees District Health Authority* (1996), Middlesbrough: Tees District Health Authority.

15  *Observer*, 10 August 1997.

16  Joint inquiry report known as 'the Broxtowe files' (1990), Nottinghamshire County Council.

17  J. S. La Fontaine (1994) *The Extent and Nature of Organised and Ritual Abuse: Research Findings*, London: HMSO.

18  *Strong Enough to Care?* (1994), Nottingham: Nottingham County Council.

19  Figures taken from a summary of epidemiological surveys quoted in *NCH Action For Children '98 Fact File*, see note 1 (this chapter).

20  Office for Standards in Education (1996) *Exclusions from Secondary Schools*, London: The Stationery Office.

21  In an influential study, *Misspent Youth* by the Audit Commission (1996), school exclusion was the factor in the lives of young people most likely to be associated with a higher level of youth crime.

22  D. Warren (1997) *Foster Care in Crisis: A Call to Professionalise the Forgotten Services*, London: National Foster Care Association.

23  Department of Health statistics, see note 3 (this chapter).

24  Ibid.

25  John Redwood was quoted in the *News of the World*, 13 August 1995.

26  *For Children's Sake (Part 2): An Inspection of Local Authority Post-Placement and Post-Adoption Services* (1997), London: Social Services Inspectorate.

27  *Better Management, Better Care*, p. 24; see note 4 (this chapter).

28  '. . . *When leaving home is also leaving care* . . .': *An Inspection of Services for Young People Leaving Care* (1997), London: Social Services Inspectorate.

29  The Home Office (1996), *The British Crime Survey*, London: HMSO.

30  Documentary on Carlton TV, January 1997.

31  N. Warner (1992), *Choosing with Care: The Report of the Committee of Inquiry into the Selection, Development and Management of Staff in Children's Homes*, London: HMSO.

32  See note 6 (this chapter).

33  This figure is quoted with the agreement of Dartington Social Research Unit in their 'Matching Needs to Services' project.

34  A number of projects with low conviction rates were described in the Audit Commission's report *Misspent Youth*, see note 21 (this chapter).

35  Reported in *Community Care*, 27 August 1981.

# 5  DOES THE COMMUNITY CARE?

1  Department of Health (1996), *Personal Social Services Local Authority Statistics*, London: HMSO.
2  W. Harbert (1994) *A Lonely Death*, London: London Borough of Brent.
3  S. Pinch (1997) *Worlds of Welfare*, London: Routledge.
4  See note 1 (this chapter).
5  Ibid.
6  *Meeting the Costs of Continuing Care* (1996), York: Joseph Rowntree Foundation.
7  L. Watson (1997) *High Hopes: Making Community Care Work*, York: Joseph Rowntree Foundation/*Community Care*.
8  N. Davies (1995) *Report of the Enquiry into the Circumstances Leading to the Death of Jonathan Newby*, Oxford: Oxfordshire Health Authority.
9  T. Kitwood and K. Bredin (1994) *Evaluating Dementia Care: The Dementia Care Mapping Method*, Bradford: Bradford University.
10  Described in A. Clarke, J. Hollands and J. Smith (1996) *Windows to a Damaged World*, London: Counsel and Care.
11  Reported in a Cornish weekly newspaper, 1997.
12  W. Boyd (1996) *Confidential Inquiry into Homicides and Suicides by Mentally Ill People* ('Boyd Report'), London: Royal College of Psychiatrists.
13  *The Report into the Care and Treatment of Martin Mursell* (1997), London: Camden and Islington Health Authority.
14  *Rampton Special Health Authority Annual Report* (1996), Retford: Rampton Hospital Authority.
15  *The Report of the Inquiry into the Care and Treatment of Christopher Clunis* (1994), presented to the Chairman of North East Thames and South East Thames Regional Health Authorities, London: HMSO.
16  C. Pierides and D. Roy (1996) *The Care Programme in West Lambeth: 3 Year Results*, London: West Lambeth Community Care Trust.
17  *London's Mental Health: The Report to the King's Fund London Commission* (1997), London: King's Fund Publishing.
18  *The Report of the Inquiry into the Treatment and Care of Gilbert Kopernick-Steckel* (1997), Croydon: Croydon Health Authority.
19  J. Reed (1992) *Review of Health and Social Services for Mentally Disordered Offenders and Others Requiring Similar Services*, London: HMSO.
20  D. Robbins (1996) *Mentally Disordered Offenders: Improving Services*, London: Social Services Inspectorate.
21  Department of Health (1991) *Hear Me: See Me: An Inspection of Services from Three Agencies to Disabled People in Gloucestershire*, London: HMSO.
22  *Adults at Risk: Procedural Guide for Professionals* (1992) Gloucester: Gloucestershire County Council, Gloucestershire Health Authority, East Gloucestershire NHS Trust and Gloucestershire Family Health Services Authority.

23  Reported in *The Economist*, 13 September 1997.
24  Baroness Cox and Lord Pearson (1995) *Made to Care*, London: The Rannoch Trust.
25  A report on the programme of 8 inspections of learning disability services was due for publication by the Social Services Inspectorate early in 1998.
26  The Health Education Authority website can be found on the Internet at http://www.hea.org.uk/
27  Department of Health (1997) *The National Treatment Outcome Research Study*, London: HMSO.
28  *Tackling Drugs Together: A Strategy for England 1995–8* (1995), London: HMSO.
29  Based on statistics in the 1990 *UK General Household Survey*, Office for National Statistics, London: HMSO.
30  S. R. Nuttall *et al.* (1994) 'Financing long-term care in Great Britain', *Journal of the Institute of Actuaries*, 121,1–68.
31  E. Holzhausen (1997) *Still Battling? The Carers Act One Year On*, London: Carers National Association.

# 8  SOMETHING SPECIAL

1  *Home Life: A Code of Practice for Residential Care* (1984), London: Centre for Policy on Ageing.
2  *A Better Home Life* (1996), London: Centre for Policy on Ageing.
3  T. Burgner (1996) *The Regulation and Inspection of Social Services*, Department of Health and Welsh Office, London: HMSO.

# 9  MORE THAN A PIECE OF PAPER

1  Department of Health (1991) *Personal Social Services Training Strategy*, London: HMSO.
2  M. Yelloly (1995) 'Professional competence and higher education' in M. Yelloly and M. Henkel (eds) *Learning and Teaching in Social Work: Towards Reflective Practice*, London: Jessica Kingsley Publishers.
3  CCETSW (1996) *Employment Survey of Newly Qualified Social Workers*, London: CCETSW.
4  P. Marsh and J. Triseliotis (1996) *Ready to Practise? Social Workers and Probation Officers: Their Training and First Year in Work*, Aldershot: Avebury Press.

# 10  THE MANAGER'S TALE

1  European Commission (1997) 'Partnership for a new organisation of work', *Supplement 4/97 to the European Union Bulletin*, Brussels: Office for Official Publications of the European Community.
2  D. Statham (1996) *The Future of Personal and Social Care*, London: National Institute of Social Work.

3  R. W. Chapman (ed.) (1980) *Boswell's Life of Johnson*, Oxford: Oxford University Press.
4  J. K. Barratt (1998) *Report of the 1997 Inquiry on 'The Trotter Affair'*, London: London Borough of Hackney.
5  J. Le Carré (1996) *The Tailor of Panama*, London: Hodder and Stoughton.

## 11  ACTS OF CHARITY

1  The quoted figures refer to losses sustained by the whole voluntary sector, not just those agencies involved in welfare.

## 12  ALL IN IT TOGETHER

1  J. Renshaw, 'Law and order', *Guardian*, 26 November 1997, Society section page 6.
2  Children's Services Project Group (1997) *Planning for Children's Services*, London: London Region Social Services Inspectorate.

# Bibliography

Adams, R. (1996) *The Personal Social Services: Clients, Consumers or Citizens?*, Harlow: Longman.

Allen of Hurtwood, Lady (1944) Letter, *The Times*, 15 July 1944.

Allen of Hurtwood, Lady (1945) *Whose Children?*, London: Allen.

Audit Commission (1986) *Making a Reality of Community Care*, London: HMSO.

Barclay Committee (1982) *Social Workers: The Roles and Tasks*, London: Bedford Square Press/National Institute for Social Work.

Beresford, P. (1994) 'Changing the culture: involving service users', in *Social Work Education*, London: Central Council for Education and Training in Social Work.

Beresford, P. and Trevillion, S. (1995) *Developing Skills for Community Care: A Collaborative Approach*, Aldershot: Arena.

Biestek, F. (1961) *The Casework Relationship*, London: Allen & Unwin.

Booth, C. (1902) *Life and Labour of the London Poor*, 17 volumes, London.

Booth, T. (1996) 'Learning difficulties', in M. Davies *The Blackwell Companion to Social Work*, Oxford: Blackwell.

Bradfield, W. (1913) *The Life of Thomas Bowman Stephenson BA, LLD, DD*, London: Charles H. Kelly.

Castle, S. and Dobson, R. (1997) 'Hit squads to tackle child abuse', *Independent on Sunday*, 19 October.

Chappell, A. (1992) 'Toward a sociological critique of the normalisation principle', *Disability, Handicap and Society*, 7(1).

Clyde, Lord (1992) *The Report of the Inquiry into the Removal of Children from Orkney in February 1991*, Edinburgh: HMSO.

Collins, J. (1995) 'Moving forward or moving back? Institutional trends in services for people with learning difficulties', in T. Philpot and L. Ward *Values and Visions: Changing Ideas in Services for People with Learning Difficulties*, Oxford: Butterworth-Heinemann.

Committee on Local Authority and Allied Personal Social Services (Seebohm Committee) (1968) *Report of the Committee on Local Authority and Allied Personal Social Services*, London: HMSO.

Cooper, J. (1983) *The Creation of the British Social Services 1962–1974*, London: Heinemann Educational.

Cormack, U. (1953) *The Welfare State*, London: Family Welfare Association.

Cresswell, J. (1997) 'Laming issues no confidence warning after Neave report', *Community Care*, 22 October.

Croft, S. and Beresford, P. (1996) 'Services users' perspectives', in M. Davies (ed.) *The Blackwell Companion to Social Work*, Oxford: Blackwell.

Curtis Committee (1946) *Report of the Care of Children Committee*, London: HMSO.

Department of Finance and Personnel (1997) *The Comprehensive Spending Review for Northern Ireland*, Belfast: Department of Finance and Personnel.

Department of Health (1989) *Caring for People: Community Care in the Next Decade and Beyond*, London: HMSO.

Department of Health (1991) *Working Together: A Guide to Arrangements for Inter-agency Co-operation for the Protection of Children from Abuse*, London: HMSO.

Department of Health (1992) *Memorandum on the Financing of Community Care Arrangements after April 1992 and on Individual's Choice of Residential Accommodation*, London: HMSO.

Department of Health (1995) *Child Protection: Messages from Research*, London: HMSO.

Department of Health (1997) *Community Care Statistics 1997: Residential Personal Social Services for Adults, England*, London: HMSO.

Ellis, K. (1993) *Squaring the Circle: User and Carer Participation in Needs Assessment*, York: Joseph Rowntree Foundation/Community Care.

Emerson, E. (1992) 'What is normalisation?', in H. Brown and H. Smith (eds) *Normalisation: A Reader for the Nineties*, London: Tavistock/Routledge.

Etherington, S. (1996) 'To the Millennium: the changing pattern of voluntary organisation', in C. Hanvey and T. Philpot (eds) *Sweet Charity: The Role of Workings and Voluntary Organisations*, London: Routledge.

Flynn, N. (1996) 'A mixed blessing? How the contract culture works', in C. Hanvey and T. Philpot (eds) *Sweet Charity: The Role and Workings of Voluntary Organisations*, London: Routledge.

Flynn, N. and Hurley, D. (1993) *The Market for Care*, London: London School of Economics.

George, V. and Wilding, P. (1985) *Ideologies and Social Welfare*, London: Routledge & Kegan Paul.

Glendinning, C. and Bewley, C. (1992) *Involving Disabled People in Community Care Planning: The First Steps*, Manchester: Department of Social Policy and Social Work, University of Manchester Press.

Goffman, E. (1962) *Asylums: Essays on the Social Situation of Mental Patients and Other Inmates*, New York: Doubleday.

Griffiths, R. (1983) *The NHS Management Inquiry*, London: HMSO.

Griffiths, R. (1988) *Community Care: Agenda for Action*, London: HMSO.

Gutch, R. (1992) *Contracting: Lessons from the USA*, London: National Council for Voluntary Organisations.

Hanvey, C. and Philpot, T. (1996a) 'Introduction', in C. Hanvey and T. Philpot (eds) *Sweet Charity: The Role and Workings of Voluntary Organisations*, London: Routledge.

Hanvey, C. and Philpot, T. (1996b) 'Survival of the fittest', *Community Care*, 30 October.

Harding, T. and Beresford, P. (eds) (1996) *The Standards We Expect: What Service Users and Carers Want from Social Services Workers*, London: National Institute for Social Work.

Harding, T. and Phillips, J. (1996) 'Providing long-term care through the market: experience in the USA', *Journal of Interprofessional Care*, 10(1).

*Henderson's Top 2000 Charities* (1995) London: Hemington Scott Publishing.

Holman, R. (1995) *The Evacuation: A Very British Revolution*, Oxford: Lion Publishing.

Hoyes, L., Jeffers, S., Lart, R., Means, R. and Taylor, M. (1993) *User Empowerment and the Reform of Community Care: An Interim Assessment*, Bristol: School for Advanced Urban Studies, University of Bristol.

Hoyes, L. and Lart, R. (1992) 'Taking care', *Community Care*, 12 February.

Jones, K. (1972) *A History of the Mental Health Services*, London: Routledge & Kegan Paul.

Kearney, B. (1992) *The Report of the Inquiry into Child Care Policies in Fife*, Edinburgh: HMSO.

Kilbrandon Report (1964) *Report of the Committee on Children and Young Persons (Scotland)*, Edinburgh: HMSO.

Laing & Buisson (1992) *Laing's Review of Private Health Care, 1992*, London: Laing & Buisson.

Laming, H. (1997), *Better Management, Better Care*, London: The Stationery Office.

McBoyle Report (1963) *Report of the Committee on the Prevention of the Neglect of Children*, Edinburgh: HMSO.

Marsh, P. (1996) 'Task-centred social work', in M. Davies (ed.) *The Blackwell Companion to Social Work*, Oxford: Blackwell.

Marsh, P. and Fisher, M. (1992) *Good Intentions: Developing Partnership in Social Services*, York: Joseph Rowntree Foundation/*Community Care*.

Martin, L. and Gaster, L. (1993) 'Community care planning in Wolverhampton', in R. Smith, L. Gaster, L. Harrison, L. Martin, R. Means and P. Thistlewaite (eds) *Working Together for Better Community Care*, Bristol: School for Advanced Urban Studies, University of Bristol.

Mayo, M. (1994) *Communities and Caring: The Mixed Economy of Welfare*, London: Macmillan.

Means, R. and Smith, R. (1994) *Community Care: Policy and Practice*, Basingstoke: Macmillan.

National Commission on the Future of the Voluntary Sector (1996) *Meeting the Challenge of Change: Voluntary Action into the 21st Century*, London: National Council for Voluntary Organisations.

Northern Ireland Council for Voluntary Action (1997) *State of the Sector*, Belfast: Northern Ireland Council for Voluntary Action.

Northern Ireland Office (1993) *Strategy for the Support of the Voluntary Sector and Community Development in Northern Ireland*, Belfast: Northern Ireland Office.

Osborne, S. P. (1994) *The Once and Future Pioneers?*, Birmingham: Aston Business School.

Parker, R. (1988) 'An historical background', in *Residential Care: The Research Reviewed*, vol. 3 of the Wagner Report, London: HMSO.

Parker, R. (1990) *Away from Home: A History of Child Care*, Barkingside: Barnardo's.

Parsloe, P. and Stevenson, O. (1993) *Community Care and Empowerment*, York: Joseph Rowntree Foundation/*Community Care*.

Peace, S., Kellaher, L. and Willcocks, D. (1997) *Re-evaluating Residential Care*, Buckingham: Open University Press.

Philpot, T. (1985) 'Puppets on a string', *Community Care*, 21 February.

Philpot, T. (1993) 'Strategic thinking', *Community Care*, 16/23 December, 22–3.

Philpot, T. (1994a) *Action for Children*, Oxford: Lion Publishing.

Philpot, T. (1994b) *Managing to Listen: A Guide to User Involvement for Mental Health Service Users*, London: King's Fund Centre.

Philpot, T. (1997) 'Strategic thinking', *Community Care*, 27 February–5 March, 26–7.

Pinker, R. (1982) 'An alternative view', in Barclay Committee, *Social Workers*, London: Bedford Square Press.

Prochaska, F. (1990) 'Philanthropy', in F. M. L. Thompson (ed.) *The Cambridge Social History of Britain, 1750–1950*, vol. 3, Cambridge: Cambridge University Press.

Richardson, J. (1995) *Purchase of Service Contracting: Some Evidence on UK Implementation*, London: National Council for Voluntary Organisations.

Russell, L., Scott, D. and Wilding, P. (1995) *Mixed Fortunes. The Funding of the Local Voluntary Sector*, Manchester: University of Manchester Press.

Schorr, A. (1992) *The Personal Social Services: An Outside View*, York: Joseph Rowntree Foundation.

Scottish Education and Scottish Home and Health Departments (1966) *Social Work and the Community*, Edinburgh: HMSO.

Scottish Office (1990) *Review of Child Care Law in Scotland: Report of a Review Group by the Secretary of State*, Edinburgh: HMSO.

Social Services Inspectorate (1991) *Care Management and Assessment: Summary of Practice Guidance: Manager's Guide, Practitioner's Guide*, London: HMSO.

Social Services Inspectorate (1997a) *A Service on the Edge: Inspection of Services for Deaf and Hard of Hearing People*, London: The Stationery Office.

Social Services Inspectorate (1997b) *For The Children's Sake (Part 2): An*

*Inspection of Local Authority Post-placement and Post-adoption Services*, London: The Stationery Office.

Social Services Inspectorate (1997c) *Inspection of Child Protection Services in Cambridgeshire*, London: Social Services Inspectorate/Department of Health.

Social Services Inspectorate/Audit Commission (1997a) *Sefton: A Report of the Review of Social Services in Sefton Metropolitan Borough Council*, Abingdon: Audit Commission Publications

Social Services Inspectorate/Audit Commission (1997b) *Stockport: A Report of the Review of Social Services in Stockport Metropolitan Borough Council*, Abingdon: Audit Commission Publications.

Townsend, P. (1986) 'Ageism and social policy', in C. Phillipson and A. Walker (eds) *Ageing and Social Policy: A Critical Assessment*, Aldershot: Gower.

Wagner, G. (1979) *Barnardo*, London: Eyre & Spottiswoode.

Wagner, G. (1988) *Residential Care: A Positive Choice. Report of the Independent Review of Residential Care*, London: HMSO.

Walker, A. (1992) 'Community care policy: from consensus to conflict', in J. Bornat, C. Pereria, D. Pilgrim and F. Williams (eds) *Community Care: A Reader*, Buckingham: Open University Press/Macmillan.

Warner, N. (1992) *Choosing with Care*, London: HMSO.

Warner, N. (1997) 'Preventing child abuse in children's homes', in S. Hayman (ed.) *Child Sexual Abuse: Myth and Reality*, London: Institute for the Study and Treatment of Delinquency.

Wolfensberger, W. and Thomas, S. (1983) *Program Analysis of Services Systems' Implementation of Normalisation Goals (PASSING): A Model of Evaluating the Quality of Human Services According to the Principles of Normalisation, Normalisation Criteria and Rating Manual*, 2nd edition, Toronto: National Institute on Mental Retardation.

Younghusband, E. (1978) *Social Work in Britain: 1950–1975: A Follow-up Study*, vol. 2, London: Allen & Unwin.

Younghusband, E. (1981) *The Newest Profession: A Short History of Social Work*, Sutton: IPC Business Press.

# Index